This Cookbook is for all
who desire good nutrition and
want to enjoy sweet treats.

The recipes use polyunsaturated fats, sugar substitutes, fresh fruits, vegetables, and carob. Many of the recipes contain zero fat and zero sugar.

My goal with this dessert book is to provide everyone with sweet treats that will not harm the human body and will provide enjoyment for the millions of people with sugar-related disease, cardiovascular disease, those with medical problems who feel deprived of their treats and for those who are strong and healthy and wish to remain so through good nutrition without deprivation of food.

May you enjoy these easy-to-make dessert recipes that feed the body and the soul with the sweetness of life itself.

—Coleen Howard

T0050578

ATTENTION: ORGANIZATIONS AND CORPORATIONS
Most Harper paperbacks are available at special quantity discounts for bulk purchases for sales promotions, premiums, or fund raising. For information, please call or write:

Special Markets Department, HarperCollins Publishers, 10 East 53rd Street, New York, New York 10022-5299. Telephone: (212) 207-7528.   Fax: (212) 207-7222.

THE DIABETIC DESSERT COOKBOOK

COLEEN HOWARD

Foreword by GEORGE SEBERG, M. D.

HARPER

An Imprint of HarperCollinsPublishers

The recipes herein are not meant to replace the advice of a licensed health care practitioner. The reader should consult his or her own physician regarding any dietary requirements or restrictions.

The nutritional values were provided by computer software from ESHA Research, Salem, Oregon. Isomalt® is a registered trademark, distributed in the United States by Palatini, Inc., U.S.A.

HARPER

An Imprint of HarperCollins*Publishers*
10 East 53rd Street
New York, New York 10022-5299

Copyright © 1997 by Coleen Howard
ISBN 978-0-06-210910-1

All rights reserved. No part of this book may be used or reproduced in any manner whatsoever without written permission, except in the case of brief quotations embodied in critical articles and reviews. For information address Harper paperbacks, an Imprint of HarperCollins Publishers.

First Harper mass market printing: January 2012
First Avon Books paperback printing: April 1997

HarperCollins® and Harper® are registered trademarks of Harper-Collins Publishers.

Printed in the United States of America

Visit Harper paperbacks on the World Wide Web at
www.harpercollins.com

10 9 8 7 6 5 4 3

If you purchased this book without a cover, you should be aware that this book is stolen property. It was reported as "unsold and destroyed" to the publisher, and neither the author nor the publisher has received any payment for this "stripped book."

This book is dedicated to my husband, Charles, who has provided the inspiration for this book and supported all my efforts in life. Because of his love and his encouragement, it is possible to share this book with you.

He deserves all the sweetness of life itself.

About the Author

Coleen Howard is a nutrition consultant who has been making and writing about candy for years. Several of her cookbooks have already been published. She lectures and teaches on current nutritional guidelines and changes in the health care field related to diabetes and other sugar diseases. She also appears on television cooking shows and radio talk shows.

Coleen was inspired to make desserts without sugar because her husband is diabetic. With the need of proper diet for diabetics in mind, she created these dessert recipes.

Millions of people are afflicted with diabetes and other diseases that require special diets. Many of these diets restrict sugar and fat altogether, or require that only small amounts be ingested. Guidelines for persons afflicted with sugar-related diseases have changed. Today, diets include natural sugars (fructose) and some polyunsaturated fats, important to a healthy, stable individual.

Desserts can be made without sugar and with healthy ingredients. The author's inspiration to produce good and fun foods for her husband brought about the creation of these desserts to be shared by all.

Through the author's knowledge and experiments, as well as her husband's willingness to taste it all, the following no- and low-sugar desserts were developed. Now all can enjoy and reap the benefits of these efforts—her recipes and his taste buds!

Foreword

As a practicing internist for the last twenty years, it has been a constant battle to find appropriate diets for treatment of the major medical maladies of our time. Diet plays a pivotal role in diabetes, heart disease, cancer and most other chronic medical problems. The medical literature is replete with different dietary regimes for every possible medical illness. The lay literature has comparable amounts of data about everything from pineapple diets to Weight Watchers. The failure or success of many diets rests upon the dedication of the dieter and the type of foods that he or she is able to ingest without exceeding certain caloric limits.

I feel that the acceptable and effective diets available in our country today have a common thread running through them. The best characteristics of all diets contain elements that are essential for weight loss in an obese individual, control of the blood sugar in a diabetic, or control of the lipids in severe hyperlipidemia. I think that a strong but neglected part of all diets is the exercise component. If a person does not change the activity level at the same time they change their intake levels, there can be no weight loss.

The common elements in all diets are what you eat, when you eat, and how you eat it. How you eat is particularly important. Sit down at a specific time. The food should be served in a reasonable manner. The amounts of food should be carefully controlled. The patient should not have the distraction of extra portions or prohibited food being readily available. It is important to make sure that the meal setting is quiet and stress-free. It should occur at the same time every day. It takes a minimum of twenty minutes to eat. It also takes twenty minutes for the brain to get the signal from the stomach that it is full. If you clock the average eating time in a busy restaurant with a stopwatch, you will find that five minutes is more the norm than twenty minutes.

But what you eat is the key in any diet. A balance must be maintained between fats, carbohydrates and proteins. Fat should constitute less than thirty percent of the diet, and carbohydrates should be high and protein low. With that in mind, it is important to modify the composition of the foods that one eats in each disease state and avoid certain types and quantities of foods. Unfortunately in America today, too many people eat fast food and other calorically empty foods that mightily contribute to a high instance of heart disease, diabetes, obesity and ongoing chronic medical problems. It is very important to make a strategic shift in the types of food products that we consume. However, I strongly feel that shifts in the diet must be made gradually by substitutions, exchanges and cross-referencing one type of food for another. These changes can be made using the available products that we have today. With minimal effort, most people can come up with a program to place themselves in a healthier eating bracket than they have previously maintained.

I am delighted to introduce a book that goes a long way to help diabetics make the transition to safe eating. With her *Diabetic Dessert Cookbook,* Mrs. Howard adds another arrow to our armament to fight off "bad eating." She takes out the simple sugars, the chemicals and the calorie-adding techniques from dessert making. She gives us an alternate choice in our diets for the psychological sweet tooth, which we all have trouble denying. She has time and taste tested each one of the recipes. I wholeheartedly endorse her efforts. With this book comes a large step in the move toward better eating for the health-conscious and for people who are on restricted diets for a multitude of medical illnesses.

George Seberg, M.D., Internist

Contents

THE DIABETIC DESSERT COOKBOOK

Introduction

Over a century ago the first case of diabetes mellitus was diagnosed. Thus began the search for the treatment, cure and management of this debilitating and life-threatening disease. The value of research has been demonstrated by the resulting constant change in diabetes management through the years. It is now possible for the diabetic to remain active and have a full, productive and long life.

Research has defined two types of diabetes, Type I and Type II. Type I requires insulin and Type II requires oral medication. In addition to medication, a program of exercise, weight control and nutrition is significant in improvement of the overall health of the diabetic.

The goal for the prevention and treatment of the acute complications of diabetes mellitus, such as hypoglycemia, short-term illnesses and exercise-related problems, renal disease, autonomic neuropathy, hypertension and cardiovascular disease, has led us to current diabetic management programs.

Many changes supporting and enhancing the quality of life have occurred through the years. Major breakthroughs in nutrition have provided less rigid diets and more options in those diets. For instance, in 1921 the diabetic was allowed ten percent protein in the daily diet. Later research raised the daily allowance to ten to twenty percent. The diet for the diabetic in 1921 was rigid. In today's world, the diabetic works on an individual basis with health care providers to use improved dietary supplements to better enjoy meals as well as provide the body with the proper nutrition.

Through research, and with today's standards, it has been found that not only does sugar play an integral part in daily nutrition, but fat content is important as well. Today there are polyunsaturated fats, and sugar and salt substitutes that allow a higher quality serving and more foods for consumption within the dietary needs of the individual. Current nutritional standards even include higher daily percentages of fructose and carbohydrate consumption. The current guidelines health care professionals follow as well as those listed by the American Diabetic Association set nutritional values on a daily basis, including calories, carbohydrates, cholesterol, fat, fiber and protein. These values are also used in the daily nutrition of the individual diabetic.

While all of us need to be aware of nutritional values, this information is of particular importance to those with diabetes, cardiovascular disease, and other sugar-related disease. Today, people are increasingly aware of food consumption and the need for good daily nutrition. The best preventative medicine we have is controlling what we eat. These recipes are to make nutritional planning more interesting and satisfying, but are not "in addition" to current food intake.

The most recent research recognizes the need for daily food consumption to be enjoyable. This is especially true for a person who feels deprived and craves certain nutrients such as sugar. For the diabetic, there is a craving for sugar. It is important for the diabetic and those with other sugar-related diseases to satisfy these cravings.

There are over three million people in the United States alone diagnosed with diabetes mellitus and many more not yet diagnosed. This does not include those with related medical complications of heart disease and hypoglycemia. My husband is one of the three million with diabetes mellitus; through him I learned about the cravings and the need to satisfy those cravings. Thus began my quest for good nutrition and enjoyment of food on a daily basis, and the result is this book.

This cookbook is for all who desire good nutrition and want to enjoy sweet treats. These dessert recipes were developed over a long period of time. They are original recipes. Each recipe has been designed with nutritional values in mind, as well as providing the sweets that we all desire and sometimes crave.

The recipes use ingredients that are friendly to the human body, including polyunsaturated fats, sugar substitutes, fresh fruits, vegetables and carob. Many of the recipes contain zero fat and zero sugar. Each recipe contains the measurement of the five main categories of nutritional values per serving. In the appendix you will find a complete analysis of each recipe.

My goal with this dessert cookbook is to provide everyone with sweet treats that will not harm the human body and will provide enjoyment for the millions of people with sugar-related disease, cardiovascular disease, those with medical problems who feel deprived of their treats and for those who are strong and healthy and wish to remain so through good nutrition without deprivation of food.

May you enjoy these easy-to-make dessert recipes that feed the body and the soul with the sweetness of life itself.

Coleen Howard

CANDIES, SQUARES, AND DESSERT BARS

Candy-Making Tips

All recipes in this book are original recipes by Coleen Howard. Each recipe has been tested to perfection.

ARTIFICIAL SWEETENER: Artificial sweetener used in these recipes is in liquid form. Granulated artificial sweeteners are acceptable. Use the same amount as noted for the liquid form. It is advisable to use granulated artificial sweeteners when used as a coating for the finished product.

CAROB: Carob is the replacement for chocolate. Melt carob as you would chocolate. Use your double boiler with hot, not boiling, water. If you do not have a double boiler, a metal bowl placed over a bowl of hot water will suffice. When carob is melted, it may form a soft ball. Cool to the point of handling the carob. Then knead in the remaining ingredients. This will not change the texture of your finished product. When the carob has melted, add the artificial sweetener. Your desserts, including truffles, will have the flavor of chocolate. If you prefer a more liquid form of melted carob, add polyunsaturated oil (one tablespoon per cup of melted carob). Add until desired liquidity is reached. Remember to change the nutritional values to include the additional oil.

You can purchase a presweetened carob. If you prefer to use presweetened carob, note any change in nutritional values. Most presweetened carob uses non-nutritional sweeteners. The recipes in this book use unsweetened carob.

COOKING STAGES: If you use a candy thermometer, cook your candy as follows:

Cold Water Stage	Equivalent Candy Thermometer Temperature
"Soft ball"	234–240°
"Hard ball"	250–269°
"Crack" or "Soft crack"	270–290°
"Hard crack" or "Brittle"	300–310°

When using a candy thermometer, cook your candy to the exact temperature as noted above. If you are cooking in altitudes over 3,000 feet (especially for creamy candies), subtract two to four degrees.

If you are using the cold water method for testing candy, drop ½ teaspoon of the cooking candy mixture into one cup of cold water. Be sure water is very cold. Let stand for approximately one minute and then check the firmness of the cooled candy with your fingers.

DIETETIC: This refers to items that can be purchased in the grocery store in the diet section. These items include canned fruits and vegetables packed in water rather than heavy sugary syrups. If you cannot find these items, then purchase the regular fruits and place them in a colander. Run cold water over the fruit to remove the sugary syrup.

EXTRACTS: Do not use artificial extracts in these recipes. They may prevent the candy from setting properly and may also alter the taste.

FRUIT: The fruits noted in the recipes are fresh fruit unless specified as dried fruit.

GRAININESS: Once a spoon is used to mix and dissolve the candy, rinse the spoon and dry. Do this often to remove any granules. Do not scrape your cooking pot. The grains will adhere to the sides of the pot. Leave them in the pot—not in your candy!

GRANOLA: Check the nutritional values on the package of granola. Some granola contains sugar. The granola in these recipes does not contain sugar.

INGREDIENTS: The ingredients for the recipes in this book are readily available in your local grocery stores and health food stores. Isomalt® (sugar substitute and hardening agent) is listed below for purchase by mail. Wherever possible, ingredients that do not contain sugar are used.

ISOMALT®: Isomalt® is a sugar substitute for specific recipes. It is a hardening agent. The remaining recipes use any liquid or granulated non-nutritional sweeteners on the market.

To make powdered Isomalt®, place the Isomalt® in a blender. Blend on highest speed until Isomalt® becomes a powder. Store in an airtight container. Use the powdered Isomalt® in all recipes calling for "powdered Isomalt®." Use Isomalt® in its original form in all other recipes.

Isomalt® may be purchased from Palatini, Inc. U.S.A., c/o Material Trans Action, Inc., 2741 N. Foundation Drive, South Bend, Indiana 46634. At the time of this publication the product was not available in retail stores.

MAPLE SYRUP: Some recipes call for "sugarless maple syrup." Check the labels carefully when purchasing sugarless maple syrup. Maple syrup is a sugar unto itself.

MARGARINE: The margarine used in these recipes is unsalted. Where salt is indicated in a recipe, a salt substitute may be used.

MEASUREMENTS: Carob is measured by placing small pieces (about the size of chocolate chips) in the measuring cup. This is for all carob (for chocolate flavor) recipes. Other items such as shredded coconut and nuts are all measured as the recipe indicates. The shredded coconut is measured after shredding a whole coconut or purchasing coconut that is already shredded. Measure chopped nuts and fruits after the chopping process.

¼ teaspoon	=	1 milliliter
½ teaspoon	=	2 milliliters
1 teaspoon	=	5 milliliters
2 teaspoons	=	10 milliliters
½ ounce	=	1 tablespoon, or 3 teaspoons, or 15 milliliters

1 ounce	= 2 tablespoons, or 6 teaspoons, or 30 milliliters
8 ounces	= 1 cup, or 16 tablespoons, or 48 teaspoons or 250 milliliters
2.2 pounds	= 1 kilogram

MOLDS: Candy molds may be used in place of pans or cookie sheets. There are many interesting and fun shapes available. You may also use candy cutters and cookie cutters for other interesting shapes.

NUTS: The nuts used in these recipes are unsalted unless salted nuts are specified.

OTHER INGREDIENTS: The items used here are no-sugar and no-salt ingredients. Use dietetic peanut butter, margarine and other ingredients. This will assure the correct nutritional value per recipe.

PAN SIZE: Use the pan size noted in each recipe. This will give you the accurate depth of the dessert for proper nutritional values.

PER SERVING SIZE: All recipes in this book are based on a per serving size of one inch by one inch squares. The depth per square is ½ to ¾ inch.

STORAGE: All desserts should be kept in a cool, dry place. The recipes in this book can be frozen for six months.

TEXTURE: The area in which you live may affect the texture of your desserts. For instance, hard candies may become sticky if you live in a hot, humid climate. The candies should all be treated as any candy made with sugar.

UTENSILS: Use nonstick pans or cookie sheets to place the cooked candy for cooling. This eliminates the use of oil. If you are using candy molds that require the use of oil, use a diabetic spray instead.

When cooking your ingredients, do NOT use a nonstick pot. When candy is poured into a pan or mold, the extra granules will stick to the pot. You do not want those granules in your completed dessert.

Citrus Candy

2 cups orange, lemon, lime or grapefruit rind, cut in 1"
   square pieces
6 cups cold water
1/8 teaspoon artificial sweetener
1 cup powdered Isomalt®

Wash the rind well. Cut away white inner skin from
rind. Cut rind in 1" squares. Put rind, water and sweetener in a 2-quart saucepan. Bring to a boil. Cook until
water and sugar substitute are completely absorbed
by rind. Once absorbed, remove from pan and place
the cooked rind on waxed paper to cool and dry.
When cool enough to handle, roll pieces in powdered
Isomalt®. Return coated pieces to waxed paper. Let
the rind dry for approximately 24 hours. Wrap individual pieces in plastic wrap. Store in refrigerator or
freezer. Yield: 24 pieces. Size: 1" square × 1/2" deep per
piece.

Nutritional Values (per piece)

Calories:	3.33	Fiber:	.136 g
Carbohydrates:	1 g	Protein:	.061 g
Cholesterol:	0 mg	Sodium:	.12 mg
Fat:	.008 g		

Coated Citrus Candy

2 cups orange, lemon, lime or grapefruit rind, cut
  in 1" square pieces
6 cups cold water
⅛ teaspoon artificial sweetener
2 cups carob

Wash the rind well. Cut away white inner skin from
rind. Cut rind in 1" squares. Put rind, water and sugar
substitute in a 2-quart saucepan. Bring to a boil. Cook
until water and sugar substitute completely absorbed
by rind. Once absorbed, remove from pan and place
the cooked rind on waxed paper to cool and dry. Let
the rind dry for approximately 24 hours. Melt carob
and sweetener in double boiler. Dip citrus candy in
melted carob. Place on waxed paper to set. Yield: 60
pieces. Size 1" square × ⅛" deep per piece.

Nutritional Values (per piece)

Calories:	19.2	Fiber:	.054 g
Carbohydrates:	2.47 g	Protein:	.586 g
Cholesterol:	.302 mg	Sodium:	.048 mg
Fat:	.835 g		

Yummy Bananas

4 cups carob
⅛ teaspoon artificial sweetener
1 cup dried, crumbled bananas

Melt carob and artificial sweetener in double boiler.
Crumble dried bananas by placing bananas between
two pieces of waxed paper. Using a rolling pin, roll
over bananas to crumble. Add crumbled bananas to
carob. Mix well. Place in a 9"×9" square pan. Cool.
Cut into 1" squares, ¾" deep. Yield: 85 pieces.

Nutritional Values (per piece)

Calories:	54.6	Fiber:	.09 g
Carbohydrates:	6.89 g	Protein:	1.63 g
Cholesterol:	.854 mg	Sodium:	.035 mg
Fat:	2.37 g		

Truffles

4 cups carob
⅛ teaspoon artificial sweetener
1 teaspoon powdered instant coffee
1 cup finely chopped peanuts

Melt carob in double boiler. Add artificial sweetener to melted carob and stir well. You may use molds for fancy-shaped truffles or place mixture in a bowl to cool. When cool enough to form a ball, form into 1" diameter balls and roll in either instant coffee or chopped peanuts (not both). Place on waxed paper. Place truffles in refrigerator for 20 minutes to set. Yield: 90 pieces.

Nutritional Values (per piece)

Calories:	57.2	Fiber:	.112 g
Carbohydrates:	5.88 g	Protein:	1.88 g
Cholesterol:	.806 mg	Sodium:	.097 mg
Fat:	3.02 g		

Coconut Delight

3 cups shredded coconut
3 large egg whites, lightly beaten
2 teaspoons rum extract
4 cups carob
⅛ teaspoon artificial sweetener

Mix 2 cups coconut and lightly beaten egg whites.
Add rum extract. Shape into 1" diameter balls. Place
on cookie sheet. Preheat oven to 350° F. Bake for 20
to 25 minutes. Coconut balls will be lightly brown.
While the coconut balls are still warm, reshape any
balls that may have lost their round shape during
baking. Cool the coconut balls. Melt carob with artificial sweetener in double boiler. Dip coconut balls
in carob. Place on waxed paper to cool. When cool
enough to handle, roll in remaining coconut. Place
in refrigerator to set. Yield: 75 pieces.

Nutritional Values (per piece)

Calories:	22.4	Fiber:	.301 g
Carbohydrates:	1.74 g	Protein:	.523 g
Cholesterol:	.181 mg	Sodium:	1.88 mg
Fat:	1.57 g		

Coconut Drops

1 cup light Philadelphia cream cheese
2 cups shredded coconut

Mix cream cheese and coconut. Drop by 1" diameter spoonfuls onto waxed paper. Refrigerate. Yield: 90 pieces.

- For a festive touch, color the coconut with food coloring before you mix with the cream cheese. Place in small paper cups in a gift box of sugarless candies for someone you love.

Nutritional Values (per piece)

Calories:	19.2	Fiber:	.271 g
Carbohydrates:	.509 g	Protein:	.291 g
Cholesterol:	2.83 mg	Sodium:	8.21 mg
Fat:	1.87 g		

Creamy Strawberries

4 cups carob
1/8 teaspoon artificial sweetener
12 ounces light Philadelphia cream cheese
2 cups crushed strawberries, fresh or frozen

Melt carob and artificial sweetener in double boiler.
Mix cream cheese and strawberries. Add to melted
carob. Mix well. Pour into a 9"×9" square pan. Let
cool and set in refrigerator for at least 2 hours. Cut
into 1" squares, ½" deep. Place in small paper cups.
Yield: 80 pieces.

Nutritional Values (per piece)

Calories:	58.7	Fiber:	.064 g
Carbohydrates:	6.66 g	Protein:	2.31 g
Cholesterol:	1.66 mg	Sodium:	25.5 mg
Fat:	2.51 g		

Fruit Surprise

½ *cup whipping cream*
1 *cup finely chopped carob*
2 *tablespoons rum extract*
½ *cup shredded coconut*
½ *cup chopped almonds*
¼ *cup chopped dried banana chips*
¼ *cup chopped dried pineapple*

Scald the cream in a 2-quart saucepan. Remove from heat. Add chopped carob. Stir until smooth. Return to heat. Let cook for 5 to 10 minutes. Add rum extract, coconut, almonds, banana chips and pineapple chips. Pour into an 8"×8" square pan. Refrigerate 6 hours before cutting. Remove from refrigerator and cut into 1" squares. Shape each square into balls 1" in diameter. Place the balls on a plate and refrigerate for 4 hours to allow candy to set. Yield: 80 pieces.

Nutritional Values (per piece)

Calories:	26.2	Fiber:	.148 g
Carbohydrates:	2.11 mg	Protein:	.643 g
Cholesterol:	2.26 mg	Sodium:	.758 mg
Fat:	1.77 g		

Rascal Raspberries

2 cups whole raspberries
4 cups carob
⅛ teaspoon artificial sweetener
1 teaspoon vanilla extract

Wash and drain raspberries. Place raspberries in a
9"×9" square pan lined with waxed paper. Melt carob
and artificial sweetener in double boiler. Add vanilla
extract. Pour mixture over raspberries. Let cool and
cut into 1" squares, ½" deep. Yield: 90 pieces.

Nutritional Values (per piece)

Calories:	49.2	Fiber:	.108 g
Carbohydrates:	5.85 g	Protein:	1.52 g
Cholesterol:	.806 mg	Sodium:	.001 mg
Fat:	2.23 g		

Crunch Bars

1 cup carob
⅛ teaspoon artificial sweetener
2 tablespoons vegetable shortening
1½ cups coarsely crumbled saltine crackers

Melt the carob, artificial sweetener and vegetable shortening in a double boiler. Stir until smooth. Add the crumbled saltine crackers. Place in a loaf pan. Press firmly. Cool. Cut into ¼" × 1" bars, ½" deep. Yield: 36 pieces.

Nutritional Values (per piece)

Calories:	80.1	Fiber:	.128 g
Carbohydrates:	10.3 g	Protein:	2.31 g
Cholesterol:	1.01 mg	Sodium:	30.1 mg
Fat:	3.33 g		

Happy Trails

4 cups carob
3 cups dry granola
3 cups dry rice cereal
1 cup chopped peanuts
1 teaspoon vanilla extract

Melt carob in double boiler. Set aside. Mix together the granola, rice and peanuts. Add to melted carob. Stir. Add vanilla extract and stir. Spread mixture evenly on a cookie sheet lined with waxed paper. Press lightly. Cool and cut into 1" squares, ½" deep. Yield: 85 pieces.

Nutritional Values (per piece)

Calories:	85.6	Fiber:	.582 g
Carbohydrates:	9.48 g	Protein:	2.59 g
Cholesterol:	.854 mg	Sodium:	7.81 mg
Fat:	4.38 g		

Raisin Clusters

1 cup carob
⅛ teaspoon artificial sweetener
½ cup raisins

Melt carob and artificial sweetener in double boiler. Remove from heat. Stir in raisins. Place by 1" diameter × ½" deep spoonfuls on waxed paper to cool. Yield: 36 pieces.

Nutritional Values (per piece)

Calories:	35.9	Fiber:	.07 g
Carbohydrates:	5.05 g	Protein:	1 g
Cholesterol:	.504 mg	Sodium:	.242 mg
Fat:	1.4 g		

Peanut Butter and Cream Cheese Kisses

½ pound carob
⅛ teaspoon artificial sweetener
12 ounces Philadelphia light cream cheese
1 cup crunchy dietetic peanut butter

Melt carob and artificial sweetener in double boiler. Mix together cream cheese and peanut butter. Roll mixture into 1" diameter balls. Dip in melted carob. Place on waxed paper to set. Stores well in refrigerator or freezer. Yield: 80 pieces.

Nutritional Values (per piece)

Calories:	36	Fiber:	.212 g
Carbohydrates:	2.4 g	Protein:	1.79 g
Cholesterol:	.975 mg	Sodium:	26 mg
Fat:	2.21 g		

Peanut Butter Cups

4 cups carob
⅛ teaspoon artificial sweetener
2 cups smooth dietetic peanut butter

Melt carob and artificial sweetener in double boiler.
Remove from heat. Pour melted carob into chocolate
molds. Fill to half full. Then add peanut butter, leaving enough room at the top to add more carob. Add
enough carob to completely cover. Refrigerate until
set, approximately 20 minutes. Cut into 1" square × ½"
deep. Yield: 80 pieces.

Nutritional Values (per piece)

Calories:	91.9	Fiber:	.422 g
Carbohydrates:	7.25 g	Protein:	3.42 g
Cholesterol:	.907 mg	Sodium:	1.09 mg
Fat:	5.85 g		

Peanut Butter-Potato Pinwheels

½ cup cold mashed potatoes (no milk or seasoning added)
⅛ teaspoon salt or salt substitute
4 cups powdered Isomalt®
½ teaspoon vanilla extract
1 cup dietetic peanut butter

To potatoes, add salt or salt substitute and 1 cup powdered Isomalt®. Beat well. Add vanilla and turn half of mixture onto board that has been lightly dusted with powdered Isomalt®. Roll into a rectangle ¼" thick. Spread with half the peanut butter. Roll up from short side, jelly roll fashion, to 1" diameter. Repeat with remaining mixture. Chill for at least 2 hours. Slice ¼" thick. Yield: 75 pieces.

Nutritional Values (per piece)

Calories:	21.7	Fiber:	.25 g
Carbohydrates:	1.1 g	Protein:	.85 g
Cholesterol:	0 mg	Sodium:	.671 mg
Fat:	1.7 g		

Chocolate Peanut Butter Fudge

2 cups finely chopped carob
⅛ teaspoon artificial sweetener
⅔ cup cold mashed potatoes (no milk or seasoning added)
½ cup dietetic peanut butter (crunchy works best)
⅛ teaspoon salt substitute

Melt carob and artificial sweetener in double boiler. Set aside. Mix together mashed potatoes, peanut butter and salt substitute. Add mixture to melted carob. Pour into a 9" × 9" square pan. Spread evenly. Cool until set. Cut into 1" squares, ½" deep. Yield: 90 pieces.

Nutritional Values (per piece)

Calories:	33.5	Fiber:	.114 g
Carbohydrates:	3.37 g	Protein:	1.12 g
Cholesterol:	.403 mg	Sodium:	.317 mg
Fat:	1.82 g		

Peanut Butter and Banana Fudge

⅔ cup cold mashed potatoes (no milk or seasoning added)
⅛ teaspoon salt substitute
⅓ cup dietetic peanut butter (crunchy works best)
¼ cup mashed, ripe bananas

Mix together the mashed potatoes and salt substitute. Add peanut butter and bananas. Press mixture into an 8" × 8" square pan. Refrigerate until set, approximately 4 hours. Cut into 1" squares, ½" deep. This is a soft fudge and so yummy. Yield: 48 pieces.

Nutritional Values (per piece)

Calories:	14.2	Fiber:	.18 g
Carbohydrates:	1.15 g	Protein:	.545 g
Cholesterol:	0 mg	Sodium:	.462 mg
Fat:	.942 g		

Peanut Butter Balls

3 cups shredded coconut
½ cup dietetic peanut butter (smooth or crunchy)
1 teaspoon vanilla extract
2 cups shredded coconut

Combine 3 cups coconut with peanut butter and vanilla extract. Mix well. Shape into 1" diameter balls. Roll balls in the 2 cups shredded coconut. Coat thoroughly. Place in pan lined with waxed paper. Chill thoroughly. Yield: 80 pieces.

Nutritional Values (per piece)

Calories:	16.4	Fiber:	.294 g
Carbohydrates:	.649 g	Protein:	.451 g
Cholesterol:	0 mg	Sodium:	.496 mg
Fat:	1.47 g		

Peanut Butter Bars

¼ cup margarine
½ teaspoon sugar substitute
2 eggs
rind of ½ lemon, grated
2 cups sifted all-purpose flour
1½ teaspoons cinnamon
1 8-ounce can salted peanuts

Cream margarine. Add sugar substitute, eggs and lemon rind. Mix well. Add flour and cinnamon. Mix well. Add peanuts and stir. Shape into bars 1" × 1½" × 1" thick. Pat firmly. Cover with waxed paper and allow to dry overnight.

Heat oven to 375° F. Bake the bars 12 to 15 minutes. Let cool. Yield: 36 pieces.

- For an additional treat, dip bars in melted carob.

Nutritional Values (per piece)

Calories:	77.5	Fiber:	.663 g
Carbohydrates:	6.7 g	Protein:	2.56 g
Cholesterol:	11.8 g	Sodium:	4.05 mg
Fat:	4.75 g		

Peanut Butter Fudge

⅔ cup cold mashed potatoes (no milk or seasoning
   added)
½ cup crunchy dietetic peanut butter
⅛ cup salt or salt substitute
4 cups powdered Isomalt®

Grease an 8" × 8" pan. Mix potatoes with peanut butter and salt. Gradually stir in Isomalt®, mixing well.
Press into greased pan. Let stand until firm. Then cut
into 1" squares, ½" deep. See if anyone can guess you
used potatoes! (No instant potatoes please. I tried it,
it doesn't work). Yield: 80 pieces.

Nutritional Values (per piece)

Calories:	10.9	Fiber:	.129 g
Carbohydrates:	.698 g	Protein:	.414 g
Cholesterol:	0 mg	Sodium:	.185 mg
Fat:	.797 g		

Friendly Dates

¾ cup finely chopped dried figs
¾ cup finely chopped dried dates
¾ cup finely chopped English walnuts
2 tablespoons grated orange rind
2 tablespoons lemon juice
60 English walnut halves

If the figs and dates are too dry, place in a bowl of hot water to moisten. Place the figs, dates and chopped walnuts in a blender. Blend well. Place mixture on a pastry board. Sprinkle with the grated orange rind and lemon juice. Knead thoroughly until well blended. Form the mixture in a long, sausage-shaped roll, 1" in diameter. Cut the roll into ¾" thick slices. Place on waxed paper. Put 1 walnut half on top of each piece of candy. Press into candy. Allow candy to dry and become firm. Store in a cool place. May be frozen. Yield: 60 pieces.

Nutritional Values (per piece)

Calories:	57.8	Fiber:	.785 g
Carbohydrates:	5.24 g	Protein:	1.09 g
Cholesterol:	0 mg	Sodium:	1.07 mg
Fat:	4.14 g		

Candied Nuts

3 cups sugar-free maple syrup
½ cup Isomalt®
½ cup water
4 cups English walnuts or pecan halves

Put maple syrup, Isomalt® and water in a heavy sauce-pan. Bring to a boil and let the mixture cook down to approximately 2 cups or until it reaches a hard crack stage. Add nuts and coat thoroughly. Pour nuts onto a cookie sheet. Separate nuts and allow to cool and dry. Break or cut into 1" squares, ¼" deep. Yield: 90 pieces.

Nutritional Values (per piece)

Calories:	40.9	Fiber:	.201 g
Carbohydrates:	4.17 g	Protein:	.636 g
Cholesterol:	0 mg	Sodium:	15.6 mg
Fat:	2.75 g		

Granola Delight

4 tablespoons margarine
4 tablespoons sugar-free maple syrup
1 cup finely chopped dates
1 cup granola
1 cup shredded coconut

Place the margarine and maple syrup in a heavy, 2-quart saucepan. Cook over low heat until margarine is melted and blended into the maple syrup. Add the chopped dates. Continue cooking and stir constantly until the dates are almost dissolved. Remove from heat. Stir in granola. Allow to cool. When cool enough to handle, roll into balls of 1" diameter and immediately roll the ball in the shredded coconut. Yield: 60 pieces.

Nutritional Values (per piece)

Calories:	31.3	Fiber:	.562 g
Carbohydrates:	3.97 g	Protein:	.358 g
Cholesterol:	0 mg	Sodium:	4.05 mg
Fat:	1.77 g		

Stuffed Dates

48 pitted dried dates
¼ cup dietetic peanut butter
½ cup chopped pecans

Place the dried dates in hot water. Set aside until dates are soft. Mix the peanut butter with the chopped pecans. Fill each date with 1 teaspoon of the peanut butter and pecan mixture. Refrigerate. Yield: 48 pieces.

- Put shredded coconut on top of stuffed date. Not only is it pretty but it tastes good, too!

Nutritional Values (per piece)

Calories:	42	Fiber:	.855 g
Carbohydrates:	7.46 g	Protein:	.603 g
Cholesterol:	0 mg	Sodium:	.376 mg
Fat:	1.54 g		

Sweet Almonds

2 cups almonds
¼ cup margarine
⅛ teaspoon artificial sweetener

Blanch almonds by dropping into boiling water for 3 to 4 minutes. Remove and drain. Remove skin from almonds. Place the margarine in a heavy iron skillet. Cook over medium heat. When margarine is melted, add the blanched almonds. Cook until the almonds are golden brown. Remove from heat. Place the almonds in a grinder or blender. Grind or blend until mixture forms a paste. Add artificial sweetener and blend. Form into 1" diameter balls. Place on waxed paper. Flatten with a spatula. Allow to cool to room temperature. Refrigerate. Yield: 80 pieces.

Nutritional Values (per piece)

Calories:	26.3	Fiber:	.353 g
Carbohydrates:	.674 g	Protein:	.744 g
Cholesterol:	0 mg	Sodium:	.378 mg
Fat:	2.47 g		

Dream Balls

1 large, ripe banana
½ pound pitted, finely chopped dates
1 cup finely chopped English walnuts
2 cups shredded coconut

Mash the banana thoroughly with a fork. Add the chopped dates. Mix thoroughly. Add the chopped English walnuts. Mix thoroughly. Form into 1" diameter balls and roll in shredded coconut. Be sure to coat thoroughly. Refrigerate 4 hours uncovered. Yield: 60 pieces.

Nutritional Values (per piece)

Calories:	25	Fiber:	.414 g
Carbohydrates:	3.59 g	Protein:	.381 g
Cholesterol:	0 mg	Sodium:	.332 mg
Fat:	1.26 g		

Sweet Sesame

1 cup sesame seeds
1/8 teaspoon artificial sweetener
1/4 teaspoon almond extract
1/2 cup raisins
20 English walnut halves

Place the sesame seeds in a blender. Blend until smooth. Turn onto a cutting board and knead in the artificial sweetener. Knead in the almond extract. Add the raisins and knead thoroughly. Pinch off small amounts and shape into 1" diameter balls. Place on waxed paper. Flatten the balls with a spatula. Place an English walnut on top of each flattened piece of candy. Refrigerate for at least 2 hours for candy to set. Yield: 20 pieces.

Nutritional Values (per piece)

Calories:	68	Fiber:	.897 g
Carbohydrates:	3.95 g	Protein:	2.39 g
Cholesterol:	0 mg	Sodium:	3.64 mg
Fat:	5.38 g		

Granola Candy

2 cups dry granola
4 tablespoons sugar-free maple syrup
1 cup shredded coconut

In a large bowl, mix the granola and maple syrup. Mix thoroughly. Granola will be sticky. Add shredded coconut and mix until granola is thoroughly coated with the coconut and easy to handle. Form into 2" diameter balls. Wrap each piece in waxed paper or colored plastic wrap. Refrigerate. Yield: 48 pieces.

Nutritional Values (per piece)

Calories:	29.9	Fiber:	.612 g
Carbohydrates:	3.5 g	Protein:	.653 g
Cholesterol:	0 mg	Sodium:	5.01 mg
Fat:	1.66 g		

Fig Sticks

4 cups fresh, whole figs
2 cups almonds
1 cup sesame seeds

Place the figs and almonds in a grinder. Grind together. Mix thoroughly. Place the mixture on waxed
paper and roll to ⅛" thick. Cut into rectangular bars
1" wide × 3" long. Place sesame seeds in the center of
each bar. Fold sides into the middle, over the sesame
seeds. Roll to 1" diameter. Cut ¾" in length. Yield: 80
pieces.

Nutritional Values (per piece)

Calories:	59.1	Fiber:	1.54 g
Carbohydrates:	8.24 g	Protein:	1.49 g
Cholesterol:	0 mg	Sodium:	2.36 mg
Fat:	2.86 g		

Coconut Sticks

4 cups fresh figs
2 cups unsalted almonds
1 cup shredded coconut

Place the fresh figs and almonds in a grinder. Grind together. Mix thoroughly. Place the mixture on waxed paper and roll ⅛" thick. Cut into rectangular bars 1" wide × 3" long. Place the shredded coconut in the center of each bar. Fold sides into the middle, over the shredded coconut. Roll until smooth and cut ½" long. Yield: 80 pieces.

Nutritional Values (per piece)

Calories:	51.6	Fiber:	1.46 g
Carbohydrates:	8.21 g	Protein:	1.03 g
Cholesterol:	0 mg	Sodium:	1.81 mg
Fat:	2.17 g		

Fruit Bars

1 1/2 pounds fresh, whole figs
1 pound pitted dates
1/2 pound raisins
1/4 pound sunflower seed kernels
1/2 pound chopped English walnuts
1/2 pound shredded coconut
2 tablespoons carob powder

Mix together the figs, dates, raisins, sunflower seed kernels and 1/4 pound chopped walnuts. Put the entire mixture through a grinder or blender. Mixture will form a paste. Set mixture aside. Place the coconut on a board. Place the ground mixture on top of the coconut. Knead the coconut into the ground mixture. Knead in the carob powder. Shape into 1" diameter × 1 1/2" long bars. Roll in remaining 1/4 pound of chopped walnuts. Refrigerate. Yield: 100 pieces.

* Make carob powder by placing carob in a blender. Blend at high speed until mixture is in a powder form.

Nutritional Values (per piece)

Calories:	66.5	Fiber:	1.45 g
Carbohydrates:	10.6 g	Protein:	.968 g
Cholesterol:	0 mg	Sodium:	1.95 mg
Fat:	2.92 g		

Apple-Raisin Surprise

¼ *cup raisins*
½ *cup apple juice*
¼ *cup pitted dates*
1 *cup finely chopped almonds*
1 *cup finely chopped cashews*
1 *cup shredded coconut*

Place the raisins in a small bowl. Add the apple juice. Be sure fruit is covered with the juice. Refrigerate overnight. Then blend the raisins, juice and dates in a blender. Be sure to mix well. Place the mixture in a bowl. Add the almonds and cashews. Mix thoroughly. Shape into 1" diameter balls and roll in shredded coconut. Refrigerate. Yield: 60 pieces

Nutritional Values (per piece)

Calories:	38.3	Fiber:	.487 g
Carbohydrates:	3.38 g	Protein:	.874 g
Cholesterol:	0 mg	Sodium:	1.55 mg
Fat:	2.65 g		

Fancy Pecans

1 pound dried figs
¼ pound pecans
¼ pound raisins
¼ pound pitted dried dates

Place the figs, pecans, raisins and dates in a grinder or blender. Once ground, place in a bowl and mix thoroughly. Then place in an 8"×8" pan. Spread in the pan with spatula or hands. Score top into 1" squares, ½" deep. Refrigerate for at least 2 hours. Cut the squares along scored lines. Yield: 75 pieces.

Nutritional Values (per piece)

Calories:	34.2	Fiber:	.799 g
Carbohydrates:	6.53 g	Protein:	.381 g
Cholesterol:	0 mg	Sodium:	.908 mg
Fat:	1.11 g		

Striped Candy Canes

1 large egg white
½ tablespoon cold water
½ teaspoon peppermint extract
2 cups powdered Isomalt®
½ tablespoon red food coloring

Combine egg white, water and peppermint extract in a bowl. Beat with an electric beater until mixture holds a peak (3 to 4 minutes). Slowly add the powdered Isomalt®. Continue beating until mixture is stiff. Place the mixture on a board that has been covered with powdered Isomalt®. Knead until smooth.

Roll half of the mixture into a long roll that is ½ the desired thickness of the candy canes. Add red food coloring to remaining mixture. Divide red mixture into 2 halves and roll very thin. Place red rolls on each side of the white roll. Hold the top of the 3 rolls. Roll so the red and white alternate like a barber pole. Cut into 7" lengths. Turn the tops down for the hook of the canes. Set aside on a rack and allow to dry thoroughly. May be frozen. Yield: 90 canes.

These candy canes are similar to those you purchase in the store!

Nutritional Values (per cane)

Calories:	5.08	Fiber:	0 g
Carbohydrates:	.105 g	Protein:	1.06 g
Cholesterol:	0 mg	Sodium:	16.6 mg
Fat:	0 g		

Old-Fashioned Candy Canes

3 cups Isomalt®
1 cup water
¾ teaspoon peppermint extract
¾ teaspoon red food coloring

Preparation: Prepare molds for hot candy by using aluminum foil. Make a trough that is ½" wide and approximately 18" long. Make another trough that is ¼" wide and approximately 18" long. The ½" trough is for the clear candy liquid. The ¼" wide trough is for the red candy liquid. Oil the troughs well with margarine or vegetable oil.

In a 4-quart heavy saucepan, combine the Isomalt® and water. Stir well. Cook to crack stage. Remove from heat and add peppermint extract. Pour ¾ of mixture into molds of aluminum foil. Add red food coloring to balance of mixture. Pour into aluminum foil mold. As soon as candy is set, place the red stripe on top of the white stripe. Cut to 7" lengths. Fold down sides of mold. Twist the strip. Turn down the tops for the hooks. Do not move until candy has completely set. Yield: 90 canes.

Nutritional Values (per cane)

Calories:	.053	Fiber:	0 g
Carbohydrates:	.014 g	Protein:	0 g
Cholesterol:	0 mg	Sodium:	.076 mg
Fat:	0 g		

Christmas Trees

¼ cup margarine
2 cups powdered Isomalt®
¼ cup light cream
3 cups shredded coconut
green food coloring
2½ cups carob
⅛ teaspoon artificial sweetener

In a 2-quart saucepan, slowly heat margarine until golden brown. Gradually stir in powdered Isomalt®, cream and coconut. Add green food coloring. Drop by tablespoonfuls onto waxed paper. Chill until easy to handle. Shape into peaks. Melt carob in double boiler. Stir in artificial sweetener. Dip the bottom half of each peak in melted carob. Place on waxed paper to cool. Measures 1" high × ¾" diameter. Yield: 80 pieces.

• You may place your coconut mixture in a Christmas tree mold. Press mixture into each Christmas tree mold and allow to cool completely. Then dip in melted carob.

Nutritional Values (per piece)

Calories:	58.1	Fiber:	.282 g
Carbohydrates:	5.15 g	Protein:	1.30 g
Cholesterol:	1.51 mg	Sodium:	.872 mg
Fat:	3.68 g		

After Dinner Mints

4 cups powdered Isomalt®
8 to 10 tablespoons whole milk
green food coloring

Place powdered Isomalt® in a bowl. Use electric mixer.
Add milk in small amounts until mixture is stiff.
Add mint flavor. Add green food coloring. Roll into
1" diameter balls and flatten with a fork dipped in
powdered Isomalt® or place in molds of your choice.
Allow to set for at least 2 hours. Yield: 60 pieces.

Nutritional Values (per piece)

Calories:	1.56	Fiber:	0 g
Carbohydrates:	.119 g	Protein:	.084 g
Cholesterol:	.346 mg	Sodium:	1.25 mg
Fat:	.085 g		

Apricot Balls

24 dried apricots
1 ½ cups shredded coconut
2 teaspoons orange juice
⅛ teaspoon artificial sweetener

Wash and dry dried apricots. Put through food chopper together with shredded coconut. Add orange juice and artificial sweetener. Blend well. Shape into 1" diameter balls. If desired, roll in shredded coconut. Yield: 60 pieces.

Nutritional Values (per piece)

Calories:	10.8	Fiber:	.324 g
Carbohydrates:	1.16 g	Protein:	.175 g
Cholesterol:	0 mg	Sodium:	.477 mg
Fat:	.7 g		

Coconut Crisps

2 cups Isomalt®
½ cup whole milk
1½ cups shredded coconut
½ teaspoon vanilla

Heat Isomalt® and milk over low heat, stirring constantly until Isomalt® is dissolved. Increase heat and cook, stirring constantly, until candy reaches a soft ball stage. Remove from heat. Stir in coconut and vanilla. Drop from a teaspoon onto a cookie sheet equal to a 1" diameter ball. Yield: 60 pieces.

Nutritional Values (per piece)

Calories:	8.4	Fiber:	.188 g
Carbohydrates:	.401 g	Protein:	.134 g
Cholesterol:	.277 mg	Sodium:	1.4 mg
Fat:	.738 g		

Coconut Rolls

¼ *cup margarine*
4 *cups powdered Isomalt*®
¼ *cup light cream*
½ *teaspoon vanilla*
1 *cup shredded coconut*

Melt margarine in a 2-quart saucepan. Add powdered Isomalt® alternately with cream and vanilla, stirring well after each addition. Beat until smooth. Sprinkle breadboard or pastry canvas with small amount of powdered Isomalt®. Turn mixture out on board and knead until smooth and glossy, about 10 minutes. Form into 1" diameter balls and roll in coconut. Yield: 60 pieces.

Nutritional Values (per piece)

Calories:	10.9	Fiber:	.031 g
Carbohydrates:	.086 mg	Protein:	.038 g
Cholesterol:	1.1 mg	Sodium:	.43 mg
Fat:	1.18 g		

Butter Crunch

1 cup margarine
1 cup Isomalt®
2 tablespoons water
1 tablespoon sugar-free maple syrup
¾ cup chopped peanuts
1 cup carob
⅛ teaspoon artificial sweetener

Melt the margarine in a 2-quart saucepan over low heat. Remove from heat. Add Isomalt®. With a wooden spoon, stir the mixture until well blended. Return to low heat. Stir rapidly until thoroughly mixed and beginning to bubble. Add water and sugar-free maple syrup. Mix well. Put in candy thermometer. Keep heat low. Stir frequently until brittle stage (approximately 15 to 20 minutes). Remove from heat at once and take out the candy thermometer.

Sprinkle peanuts over surface and quickly mix in. Pour onto a cookie sheet. With a spatula, spread ¼" thick. Cool to room temperature. As crunch cools, loosen from sheet with spatula 2 or 3 times. Melt the carob and artificial sweetener in a double boiler. Remove from water. Stir well. Spread half of melted carob evenly over crunch. Set aside until firm. Turn onto waxed paper or another cookie sheet carob side down. Spread remaining melted carob evenly. Both sides will be coated. When firm, break candy into pieces of 1" square. Store in lightly covered container in a cool place. Yield: 80 pieces.

Nutritional Values (per piece)

Calories:	28.4	Fiber:	.095 g
Carbohydrates:	.348 g	Protein:	.339 g
Cholesterol:	0 mg	Sodium:	.322 mg
Fat:	2.96 g		

Cherry Fudge

1 1/3 tablespoons margarine
2 teaspoons grated orange rind, as desired
1 cup thin cream
3 cups Isomalt®
3/8 teaspoon cream of tartar
3 tablespoons orange juice
1 teaspoon lemon juice
2/3 cup chopped English walnuts
1 3-ounce can or jar of red maraschino cherries

Melt margarine in a 2-quart heavy saucepan. Remove from heat. Add orange rind. Blend thoroughly. Add cream, Isomalt®, cream of tartar and orange juice. Blend thoroughly. Place over low heat. Stir until Isomalt® is dissolved and mixture is boiling gently. Cover. Cook 3 minutes. Remove cover. If crystals form on sides of pan during the cooking process, remove with damp cloth wrapped around tines of a fork. Stir occasionally to soft ball stage. Because this is a very soft fudge, it must be cooked at this low temperature.

Remove from heat. Cool at room temperature until lukewarm. Add lemon juice and nuts. Beat until thick and creamy. This candy requires lots of beating. Spread evenly in a 9"×9" pan. Cool. Cut in 1" square × ½" deep pieces. Cut red petals from glossy outside peel of cherries. Use three petals to form a flower on each piece of candy. Yield: 90 pieces.

Nutritional Values (per piece)

Calories:	34.6	Fiber:	.043 g
Carbohydrates:	.651 g	Protein:	.231 g
Cholesterol:	.992 mg	Sodium:	1.28 mg
Fat:	3.56 g		

Cherries à la Fudge

4 envelopes unflavored gelatin
½ cup Isomalt®
1½ cups boiling water
2 cups carob
2 cups chopped maraschino cherries

Use a heavy 4-quart saucepan. Mix gelatin with Iso-malt®. Add boiling water and stir until gelatin is completely dissolved. Add carob, and stir with a wire whip over low heat until carob is melted and thoroughly blended. Remove from heat. Add maraschino cherries. Mix well. Pour into an 8"×8" square pan. Cool. Cut into 1" squares, ½" deep. Yield: 80 pieces.

Nutritional Values (per piece)

Calories:	33.5	Fiber:	0 g
Carbohydrates:	4.53 g	Protein:	1.13 g
Cholesterol:	.454 mg	Sodium:	10.9 mg
Fat:	1.25 g		

Creamy Fudge

1 3-ounce package light Philadelphia cream cheese
⅛ teaspoon artificial sweetener
½ teaspoon almond extract
1½ cups chopped almonds
dash of salt or salt substitute

With electric mixer, beat cream cheese until soft and smooth. Slowly blend in artificial sweetener, extract, nuts, and salt or salt substitute. Pour into an 8"×8" pan. Chill until firm. Cut into 1" squares, ½" deep. Yield: 64 pieces.

Nutritional Values (per piece)

Calories:	19.1	Fiber:	.291 g
Carbohydrates:	.668 g	Protein:	.797 g
Cholesterol:	.234 mg	Sodium:	8.3 mg
Fat:	1.59 g		

Walnut Fudge

3 cups carob
¼ teaspoon artificial sweetener
1 14-ounce can sweet condensed milk (not evaporated milk)
1 cup chopped walnuts
1½ teaspoons vanilla extract
48 walnut halves

In a heavy 2-quart saucepan, combine the carob, artificial sweetener and condensed milk. Cook over low heat until carob is completely melted. Remove from heat. Add chopped walnuts and vanilla extract. Stir until completely mixed. Pour into a 9"×9" square pan. Chill in refrigerator until almost firm. Score the top of the fudge into squares 2"×½" deep. Place a walnut half on the top of each square. Chill until firm. Finish cutting into squares. Yield: 48 2"-square pieces.

- Can be made into smaller pieces. If cut to 1" squares, lower nutritional values by 50 percent.

Nutritional Values (per piece)

Calories:	137	Fiber:	.302 g
Carbohydrates:	13.5 g	Protein:	3.72 g
Cholesterol:	3.94 mg	Sodium:	11.2 mg
Fat:	7.97 g		

Almond Delight

2 cups blanched almonds
2 cups powdered Isomalt®
Rind of ½ lemon
2 egg whites

Grind almonds very fine through a food grinder or blender. Nuts should be the consistency of dry, white sugar. When you grind the nuts, be sure the nuts are dry. If nuts seem moist and oily, spread them over a shallow pan and dry them in a slow oven, 300° F, before grinding. Put the ground almonds in a large mixing bowl, and stir in Isomalt® and lemon rind. Pound hard with the handle of a wooden spoon. Pound about 5 to 7 minutes to get all the flavor mixed through. Add unbeaten egg whites and knead. Place in an 8"×8" square pan and refrigerate. Cut into 1" squares, ½" deep. Yield: 60 pieces.

Nutritional Values (per piece)

Calories:	28.9	Fiber:	.474 g
Carbohydrates:	.909 g	Protein:	1.09 g
Cholesterol:	0 mg	Sodium:	2.15 mg
Fat:	2.54 g		

Nut Crunch

1 ¼ cups Isomalt®
¾ cup margarine
¼ cup water
½ cup unblanched almonds
½ teaspoon baking soda
½ cup blanched almonds
⅓ cup carob
⅛ teaspoon artificial sweetener
½ cup finely chopped blanched almonds

In a heavy saucepan mix Isomalt®, margarine, water and unblanched almonds. Boil mixture to brittle stage. Stir occasionally. Stir in baking soda and the blanched almonds. Pour into an 8" × 8" square pan, ¾" deep. Melt carob in double boiler. Stir in artificial sweetener and mix well. Spread sweetened carob evenly on top of candy. Sprinkle with finely chopped nuts. Cool. Break into 1" square pieces. Yield: 80 pieces.

Nutritional Values (per piece)

Calories:	35.3	Fiber:	.204 g
Carbohydrates:	1.12 g	Protein:	.594 g
Cholesterol:	.085 mg	Sodium:	.315 mg
Fat:	3.32 g		

Pralines

2 cups Isomalt®
1 teaspoon baking soda
1 cup buttermilk
pinch of salt or salt substitute
2 tablespoons margarine
2⅓ cups pecan halves
64 perfect pecan halves (unbroken)

In a large kettle (about 8 quarts), combine Isomalt®, baking soda, buttermilk and salt or salt substitute. Cook over high heat 5 minutes, being sure to stir frequently and to scrape bottom and crevices of kettle. Cook to 234° F on a candy thermometer. Remove from heat. Add margarine and 2⅓ cups pecan halves. Cook, stirring continuously to soft ball stage. Remove and let stand just a minute or 2. Then with a spoon, beat until thickened and creamy. Immediately drop by 2" tablespoonfuls onto waxed paper or a cookie sheet. Dot with perfect pecans. Press pecan into each piece of candy. Yield: 64 pieces.

Nutritional Values (per piece)

Calories:	39.2	Fiber:	.24 g
Carbohydrates:	1.13 g	Protein:	.531 g
Cholesterol:	.134 mg	Sodium:	23.7 mg
Fat:	3.89 g		

Date Roll

8 cups Isomalt®
1 cup heavy cream
1 cup dates
1 cup chopped English walnuts

Cook Isomalt® and cream in a heavy 2-quart saucepan until mixture comes to a boil. Add the dates. Cook until mixture reaches the soft ball stage. Remove from heat. Beat the mixture in the saucepan until creamy. Add the English walnuts and pour onto a damp cloth and mold into a roll 1" in diameter. Keep in cloth in the refrigerator overnight. Remove the candy from the cloth and slice ¾" thick. Yield: 60 pieces.

Nutritional Values (per piece)

Calories:	34.7	Fiber:	.314 g
Carbohydrates:	2.66 g	Protein:	.427 g
Cholesterol:	5.43 mg	Sodium:	1.78 mg
Fat:	2.72 g		

English Toffee

2 cups Isomalt®
1 ½ cups margarine
2 tablespoons water
2 cups blanched almonds
½ cup grated carob

Combine the Isomalt®, margarine and water in a heavy 2-quart saucepan. Cook over low heat so mixture will not burn. Cook until margarine is melted. Stir mixture occasionally. Add the almonds. Continue cooking slowly without stirring to 280° or to a hard crack stage. Pour into a shallow pan or onto a cookie sheet to ½" thickness. Sprinkle with the grated carob. Break into 1" square pieces. Yield: 80 pieces.

Nutritional Values (per piece)

Calories:	57.9	Fiber:	.338 g
Carbohydrates:	1.52 g	Protein:	.942 g
Cholesterol:	.113 mg	Sodium:	.484 mg
Fat:	5.58 g		

Sweet Nuts

1 cup Isomalt®
¼ cup water
1 teaspoon vanilla
1 cup chopped English walnuts

Boil Isomalt® and water until mixture threads from
a spoon or reaches a hard crack stage. Remove from
heat. Add vanilla and English walnuts. Stir well. Pour
onto a cookie sheet to ½" deep. Spread out and allow
to cool completely. Break or cut into 1" square pieces.
Yield: 100 pieces.

- Other nuts may be used, such as almonds, cashews
  or peanuts.

Nutritional Values (per piece)

Calories:	6.51	Fiber:	.045 g
Carbohydrates:	.184 g	Protein:	.143 g
Cholesterol:	0 mg	Sodium:	.101 mg
Fat:	.619 g		

Potato Bon Bons

6 potatoes
1 teaspoon vanilla
1 cup powdered Isomalt®
2 cups carob

Peel potatoes and boil. Pour off water and mash potatoes thoroughly. Add vanilla. Mix thoroughly. Add powdered Isomalt®. Mix well. Mixture will hold its shape. Shape mixture into 1" diameter balls and place on a cookie sheet. Place carob in double boiler and melt. Dip each potato ball in melted carob. Place on waxed paper to cool. Yield: 75 pieces.

Nutritional Values (per piece)

Calories:	27.3	Fiber:	.141 g
Carbohydrates:	4.24 g	Protein:	.748 g
Cholesterol:	.302 mg	Sodium:	.541 mg
Fat:	.842 g		

Cinnamon Bon Bons

1 ½ cups Isomalt®
½ cup evaporated milk
1 tablespoon margarine
½ teaspoon cream of tartar
¼ teaspoon salt or salt substitute
1 teaspoon vanilla
1 cup cinnamon
1 cup chopped English walnuts

Cook Isomalt®, milk, margarine, cream of tartar and salt or salt substitute to boiling point, stirring constantly. Continue cooking, stirring occasionally until the mixture forms a soft ball. Remove from heat. Cool to lukewarm. Add vanilla. Beat until creamy and stiff. Shape with fingers into 1" diameter balls. Then shape each ball to resemble potatoes. Roll in cinnamon. Insert 3 pieces of walnuts in each piece of candy to look like the "eyes" of a potato. Yield: 80 pieces.

Nutritional Values (per piece)

Calories:	37.9	Fiber:	.2 g
Carbohydrates:	4.44 g	Protein:	1.04 g
Cholesterol:	.341 mg	Sodium:	2.5 mg
Fat:	1.86 g		

Cream Delight

2 cups carob
1/8 teaspoon artificial sweetener
1/4 cup heavy whipping cream

Melt the carob and artificial sweetener in a double boiler. Remove the top portion of the double boiler that contains the carob and set aside. Heat the whipping cream in a separate saucepan until boiling. Gradually pour the boiling cream into the melted carob, beating constantly. Candy will become dark and appear glossy. Place the candy back on top of double boiler. Cook over medium heat. Stir constantly until candy is very thick. Remove from heat. Cool candy until it can be handled. Place on waxed paper and spread to 1/2" thick. Cut in 1" squares or use candy cutters or molds. Yield: 60 pieces.

Nutritional Values (per piece)

Calories:	25.8	Fiber:	0 g
Carbohydrates:	2.62 g	Protein:	.723 g
Cholesterol:	1.74 mg	Sodium:	.373 mg
Fat:	1.41 g		

Cocoa Balls

¾ cup cocoa
1 ¾ cups powdered Isomalt®
1 cup chopped walnuts or pecans
½ cup sweet condensed milk
1 tablespoon vanilla

Mix ½ cup cocoa and 1 ½ cups powdered Isomalt®.
Add chopped walnuts or pecans and mix thoroughly.
Add condensed milk and vanilla. Shape into 1" diameter balls. Combine the remaining powdered Iso-
malt® and cocoa in a separate bowl. Roll the balls in
the mixture until completely coated. Chill. Yield: 75
pieces.

Nutritional Values (per piece)

Calories:	19.5	Fiber:	.36 g
Carbohydrates:	1.87 g	Protein:	.453 g
Cholesterol:	.693 mg	Sodium:	2.79 mg
Fat:	1.37 g		

Buckeyes

½ cup margarine
1 pound peanut butter
4 cups powdered Isomalt®
1 cup carob chips

Cream together the margarine and peanut butter. Add powdered Isomalt® gradually and blend. The mixture will be crumbly. Shape into 1" diameter balls. Place a toothpick in each ball. Melt the carob in a double boiler. Dip each ball in the melted carob. Place on waxed paper. Chill until firm. Yield: 75 pieces.

Nutritional Values (per piece)

Calories:	61.2	Fiber:	.399 g
Carbohydrates:	2.63 g	Protein:	2.1 g
Cholesterol:	.242 mg	Sodium:	1.06 mg
Fat:	5.06 g		

Almond Balls

1 package dry yeast
¼ cup warm water
1 cup scalded whole milk (no canned milk, please!)
1 teaspoon artificial sweetener
⅓ cup margarine
½ teaspoon salt substitute
4 cups sifted all-purpose flour
3 large eggs, well beaten
¼ cup melted margarine
1 cup chopped almonds

Preheat oven to 300° F. Place the yeast in the warm water. Set aside. In a 1-quart heavy saucepan, scald the milk. Blend in the artificial sweetener, ⅓ cup margarine and the salt substitute. Stir well and continue cooking until the artificial sweetener is dissolved. Remove from heat. Add the eggs and yeast mixture. Pour into a large bowl and add the flour. Beat well. Place the mixture on a floured board and knead until smooth. Shape into a large ball. Place in a bowl and cover with a cloth. Let stand until mixture rises to double its size. Punch it down and let it rise again to twice its size. Then shape the dough into 1" diameter balls. Melt a ¼ cup of margarine. Place the melted margarine in a bowl. Place the chopped almonds in another bowl. Dip the balls into the melted margarine and then into the almonds. Coat well. Place on a cookie sheet. Cook in the oven for 15 to 20 minutes. Remove and place on waxed paper to cool. Yield: 75 pieces.

Nutritional Values (per piece)

Calories:	72.2	Fiber:	.631 g
Carbohydrates:	9.62 g	Protein:	2.08 g
Cholesterol:	7.63 mg	Sodium:	4.61 mg
Fat:	2.9 g		

Sweet Fruit

½ cup dried prunes
½ cup dried apricots
½ cup raisins
½ cup chopped cashew nuts
½ cup artificial sweetener

Rinse the prunes, apricots and raisins thoroughly.
Let dry completely. Chop the prunes, apricots and
raisins into very fine pieces. A food processor is faster;
otherwise, use a sharp knife on a wooden cutting
board. Mix the chopped nuts and fruit together. Shape
into 1" diameter balls. Place artificial sweetener in
another bowl. Roll the small balls in powdered artificial sweetener. Place on waxed paper to dry. Yield:
50 pieces.

Nutritional Values (per piece)

Calories:	18.4	Fiber:	.329 g
Carbohydrates:	3.19 g	Protein:	.338 g
Cholesterol:	0 mg	Sodium:	.499 mg
Fat:	.661 g		

Date Balls

3 tablespoons margarine
2 eggs, well beaten
2/3 cups Isomalt®
1 cup chopped dates
2 cups dry rice cereal
1 cup chopped English walnuts
1 teaspoon vanilla extract
1 cup shredded coconut

In a heavy 2-quart saucepan melt the margarine. Set aside. In a bowl, beat the eggs and Isomalt® together. Add the chopped dates. Pour this mixture into the saucepan with the melted margarine. Cook over low heat, stirring constantly, until the mixture is very thick. Remove from heat. Add rice cereal, nuts and vanilla extract. Allow mixture to cool to lukewarm, or until it can be handled comfortably. Form into 1" balls. Roll the balls in the shredded coconut. Refrigerate to set. Yield: 80 pieces.

Nutritional Values (per piece)

Calories:	27.5	Fiber:	.338 g
Carbohydrates:	2.7 g	Protein:	.41 g
Cholesterol:	5.33 mg	Sodium:	5.76 mg
Fat:	1.83 g		

Candied Prunes

80 dried, pitted prunes
1 cup water
¼ cup cider vinegar
2 sticks cinnamon
¼ teaspoon mint extract

In a heavy 4-quart saucepan cook the prunes, water, vinegar and cinnamon sticks. Bring the mixture to a boil. Continue boiling until the prunes are tender. Remove from heat. Add the mint extract. Stir well. Let stand for 12 hours in the refrigerator. Drain prunes. Keep in a cool, dry place. Yield: 80 pieces.

Nutritional Values (per piece)

Calories:	13.7	Fiber:	.524 g
Carbohydrates:	3.6 g	Protein:	.148 g
Cholesterol:	0 mg	Sodium:	.234 mg
Fat:	.029 g		

Vanilla Raisin Clusters

1 cup carob
⅛ teaspoon artificial sweetener
1 teaspoon vanilla extract
2 cups raisins

In a double boiler melt the carob. Remove from heat. Add the artificial sweetener and vanilla extract. Stir well. Add raisins. Drop by 2" square shaped spoonfuls onto waxed paper or into candy cups. Allow to cool thoroughly. Yield: 60 pieces.

Nutritional Values (per piece)

Calories:	32.5	Fiber:	.168 g
Carbohydrates:	5.92 g	Protein:	.718 g
Cholesterol:	.302 mg	Sodium:	.581 mg
Fat:	.854 g		

Filled Fruit

12 dried apricots
1 3-ounce package light Philadelphia cream cheese
¼ cup unsalted margarine
1 teaspoon vanilla extract
⅛ teaspoon artificial sweetener

Place apricots in scalding water. Let soak until soft.
Remove and let dry on a wire rack. While fruit is dry-
ing, make cream cheese filling by mixing together
the cream cheese, margarine and vanilla extract. Add
the artificial sweetener. Mix well. Place 1 teaspoon of
mixture in the center of each apricot. Yield: 12 pieces.

Nutritional Values (per piece)

Calories:	53.1	Fiber:	.465 g
Carbohydrates:	3.15 g	Protein:	1.39 g
Cholesterol:	1.25 mg	Sodium:	42.8 mg
Fat:	3.9 g		

Orange Sticks

⅓ cup orange juice
⅓ cup dry rolled oats
⅓ cup margarine
2 cups powdered Isomalt®
3 tablespoons cocoa
⅔ cup chopped walnuts
⅔ cup raisins
⅔ cup shredded coconut
¼ teaspoon ground nutmeg
¼ teaspoon ground cinnamon

In a large bowl, mix the orange juice and rolled oats. Let mixture set for 1 hour. Then place the margarine in a small saucepan. Melt over low heat. Set aside. Add the powdered Isomalt®, cocoa, walnuts, raisins, shredded coconut, nutmeg, cinnamon and margarine to the bowl containing the orange juice and rolled oats mixture. Stir well. Place in the refrigerator for at least 1 hour. Remove and form into sticks ¼" wide × ½" long × ¾" thick. Place on waxed paper or wire rack to dry. Yield: 75 pieces.

Nutritional Values (per piece)

Calories:	24.3	Fiber:	.219 g
Carbohydrates:	2.04 g	Protein:	.44 g
Cholesterol:	.048 mg	Sodium:	4.37 mg
Fat:	1.76 g		

Pumpkin Squares

1 cup cooked and mashed pumpkin
¼ teaspoon pumpkin pie spice
1 3-ounce package cream cheese
2 cups powdered Isomalt®

Cook pumpkin until partially firm. If you overcook the pumpkin, your candy will not be firm. Mash pumpkin well. The pumpkin will still hold its shape. Place pumpkin, pumpkin pie spice and cream cheese in a bowl. Blend well. Add powdered Isomalt® ½ cup at a time and stir well. Mixture will be thick. Place in an 8"×8" square pan. Refrigerate overnight. Cut into 1" squares, ½" deep. Yield: 80 pieces.

Nutritional Values (per piece)

Calories:	1.57	Fiber:	.028 g
Carbohydrates:	.191 g	Protein:	.172 g
Cholesterol:	.187 mg	Sodium:	6.4 mg
Fat:	.003 g		

Bon Bons

2 cups carob
1 teaspoon artificial sweetener
1 pint ice milk
80 small candy paper cups

Melt carob in a double boiler. Remove from heat. Add artificial sweetener and mix well. Cool to the point mixture can be spooned into paper cups. Fill each cup half full. Add small scoop of ice milk. Spoon more carob mixture over the top of the ice milk. Be sure mixture covers the ice milk. Immediately place in the freezer. Yield: 80 pieces.

* Be sure ice milk is frozen solid. If not, the ice milk will melt before you can finish spooning the melted carob over the top and placing in the freezer.

Nutritional Values (per piece)

Calories:	31.4	Fiber:	.003 g
Carbohydrates:	3.86 g	Protein:	.968 g
Cholesterol:	.916 mg	Sodium:	2.81 mg
Fat:	1.39 g		

Frosted Fruit

45 strawberries
1 egg white
2 tablespoons water
1 cup powdered Isomalt®

Wash strawberries and let dry. Place egg white and water in bowl. Beat lightly. Place the powdered Isomalt® in another bowl. Dip strawberries in egg white mixture. Then dip in powdered Isomalt®. Repeat to thicken the coating. Place on a baking sheet lined with waxed paper. Allow to dry thoroughly. Store in airtight container in the refrigerator. Yield: 45 pieces.

- Other fruits may be used. If a fruit such as dates or prunes are used, the fruit can be dipped and placed on a cookie sheet lined with cooking paper. Then place in an oven heated to 170° until dry. Remove from oven and cool. Store in airtight container in the refrigerator.

Nutritional Values (per piece)

Calories:	3.7	Fiber:	.154 g
Carbohydrates:	.721 g	Protein:	.203 g
Cholesterol:	0 mg	Sodium:	2.32 mg
Fat:	.037 g		

Dipped Pecans

5 cups powdered Isomalt®
½ cup margarine
1 egg white, stiffly beaten
1½ teaspoons vanilla extract
2 cups carob
1 teaspoon artificial sweetener
80 pecan halves

Combine 2½ cups powdered Isomalt® with margarine in a bowl. Combine the remaining 2½ cups powdered Isomalt® with stiffly beaten egg white in another bowl. Add the contents from the first bowl to the egg white mixture in the second bowl. Cream mixture together. Add vanilla extract. Knead until candy is light and creamy. Roll into a ball. Cover with waxed paper. Store in airtight container in the refrigerator for 24 hours to ripen. Remove and roll into 1" diameter balls. Melt carob and artificial sweetener in double boiler. Dip balls in melted carob. Place on cookie sheet to cool. While cooling, flatten with pecan half on each ball. Yield: 80 pieces.

Nutritional Values (per piece)

Calories:	55.3	Fiber:	.125 g
Carbohydrates:	3.62 g	Protein:	1.13 g
Cholesterol:	.454 mg	Sodium:	1.22 mg
Fat:	4.21 g		

Pretzels

4 cups carob chips
2 cups sifted cocoa

In a double boiler, melt the carob. Place in a pastry decorating bag. Squeeze out in a pretzel design onto a sheet of waxed paper in 1" diameter, ⅛" thick. Let set. Once set, dip in sifted cocoa. Place again on waxed paper to dry. Keep in a well sealed container away from heat and moisture. Yield: 60 pieces.

Nutritional Values (per piece)

Calories:	71.6	Fiber:	0 g
Carbohydrates:	8.3 g	Protein:	2.25 g
Cholesterol:	1.21 mg	Sodium:	0 mg
Fat:	3.33 g		

OTHER
SWEET TREATS

Treat-Making Tips

This section contains wonderful diabetic treats that are not candy, but do feed the soul and take care of that marvelous "sweet tooth" in a healthy and satisfying way. If you desire to make large batches of any recipe in this section, simply increase the amounts used in each recipe to suit your needs. This is especially easy and helpful for serving large groups.

When you are using the ingredients in these recipes, you will find that everyday items are used There is nothing exotic in these recipes. The results can be exotic in their appeal and taste, however.

Below are some hints when using the ingredients:

CAKE FLOUR: You may use cake flour in your recipes rather than bleached or unbleached flour where "flour" is called for. However, cake flour will change the nutritional values. When a recipe calls for "cake flour," please use that particular flour in that recipe and do not substitute an all-purpose white flour.

DIABETIC OR NO-SUGAR INGREDIENTS: When called for, please use the specified diabetic or no-sugar ingredient. Any substitution will change the nutritional values.

FAT CONTENT: The nutritional values note fat content per recipe. This is the *total* fat content and it includes saturated fat, polyunsaturated fat, and monounsaturated fat.

FLOUR: Flour used herein is an all-purpose white flour. You may use either bleached or unbleached flour. This is your choice and will not change the taste of your recipe. Flour measurements are sifted measurements.

NUTRITIONAL VALUES: Nutritional values are given on the specific recipe with the specific ingredients. Any change of ingredients will change the nutritional values.

POLYUNSATURATED OIL: Any oil used in these recipes is polyunsaturated oil to give the best for diabetic needs and healthy eating.

SUGAR SUBSTITUTE: The recipes in this section that call for sugar substitute use granulated or powdered sugar substitutes. Do not use liquid sugar substitutes. Using the same measurement as a granulated or powdered sugar substitute, your recipe will be too sweet.

Cakes

White Frosting

1 8-ounce package Philadelphia light cream cheese
¼ cup plain yogurt
1 teaspoon vanilla extract

Place the cream cheese in a small bowl. Beat until smooth. Add the plain yogurt and vanilla extract. Beat until smooth and thick. Yield: 2 cups of frosting.

To flavor white frosting use any of the following:
  ¼ cup shredded coconut
  ⅓ cup carob powder
  3 tablespoons dry buttermilk
  Any flavor of extract: almond, orange, lemon, rum, peppermint
  Any of your favorite fruits, chopped fine: strawberries, cherries, blueberries, oranges, lemons, apples, tangerines, etc.
  Use your imagination and enjoy a variety of flavors on your favorite cake.

Nutritional Values (2 cups)

Calories:	234	Fiber:	0 g
Carbohydrates:	12.6 g	Protein:	35.5 g
Cholesterol:	41 mg	Sodium:	1406 mg
Fat:	.11 g		

Cherry Cheesecake

1 Graham Cracker Crust (page 134)
1 13-ounce can evaporated skim milk
2 tablespoons cornstarch
¼ cup sugar substitute
1 3-ounce package Philadelphia light cream cheese
¼ cup pure lemon juice
1 ½ teaspoons vanilla extract
1 1-pound can unsweetened cherries with juice
2 tablespoons cornstarch
2 tablespoons sugar substitute

Prepare the graham cracker crust and place in a 9" pie pan. Set aside. In a small saucepan, cook the evaporated skim milk and cornstarch until thick. Remove from heat and add ¼ cup sugar substitute. Stir well. Set aside to cool. In a small bowl, place the cream cheese and beat well. Add the mixture from the small saucepan. Beat well. Add the lemon juice and vanilla extract. Beat until well blended. Pour into the graham cracker crust. Place in the refrigerator for 2 hours. While cooling, prepare cherry topping. Drain the cherries but save the cherry juice. Place the cherry juice and cornstarch in a small saucepan. Cook over medium heat, stirring constantly. Mixture will become thick and clear. Add the cherries and the 2 tablespoons sugar substitute. Stir well. Set aside to cool. When cool, spread over the cream cheese. Refrigerate for 1 hour. Yield: 10 pieces.

Nutritional Values (per serving)

Calories:	66.3	Fiber:	.416 g
Carbohydrates:	12 g	Protein:	4.37 g
Cholesterol:	2.82 mg	Sodium:	96.8 mg
Fat:	.129 g		

Blueberry Cake

3 large eggs
1/2 cup unsalted margarine
1 cup pure orange juice
2 1/2 cups cake flour
1 teaspoon baking soda
2 teaspoons baking powder
1 cup shredded coconut
1 cup fresh or frozen blueberries (thawed and drained)

Preheat oven to 350° F. In a large bowl mix the eggs, margarine and orange juice. Beat well. Add the cake flour, baking soda and baking powder. Beat well. Stir in the coconut and blueberries. Mix well with a spoon. Place the mixture in a nonstick 9" × 13" cake pan. Bake 25 to 30 minutes. When cool, frost with White Frosting (page 93). Yield: 32 pieces.

Nutritional Values (per serving)

Calories:	68.6	Fiber:	.684 g
Carbohydrates:	7.96 g	Protein:	1.47 g
Cholesterol:	20 mg	Sodium:	19.8 mg
Fat:	3.53 g		

Applesauce-Pineapple Cake

2 cups dietetic canned applesauce
2 cups dietetic canned crushed pineapple
1 cup unsalted margarine, melted
1 sugar-free yellow cake mix
1½ cups chopped English walnuts

Preheat oven to 350° F. In a nonstick 9" × 13" cake pan, place the ingredients as follows: Spread the applesauce on the bottom of the cake pan. Spread evenly. On top of the applesauce, pour the crushed pineapple and spread evenly but do not mix. On top of the pineapple, place the melted margarine. On top of the margarine, place the yellow cake mix and cover evenly. Do not mix. On top of the yellow cake mix, spread the English walnuts. Bake for 60 minutes. Remove to a wire rack to cool. Frost with White Frosting (page 93). Yield: 32 2" square pieces.

Nutritional Values (per serving)

Calories:	105	Fiber:	.544 g
Carbohydrates:	9.58 g	Protein:	1.27 g
Cholesterol:	.177 mg	Sodium:	84 mg
Fat:	7.29 g		

Vanilla Cake

½ cup diet margarine
¾ cup sugar substitute
2 teaspoons vanilla extract
⅓ cup egg whites
2 cups cake flour
2 teaspoons baking powder
2 tablespoons instant dry milk
½ cup lukewarm water
½ cup slivered almonds

Preheat oven to 350° F. In a large bowl, cream together the margarine, sugar substitute, and vanilla extract. Add the egg whites and beat well. In a separate small bowl, mix together with a fork the flour, baking powder and dry milk. Add the dry mixed ingredients to the large bowl. Mix well. Add the lukewarm water and beat well. Place the batter in a 9"×9" square nonstick cake pan. Sprinkle the slivered almonds on top of the batter. Bake for 30 to 35 minutes. Place on a wire rack to cool. Cut into 2" squares. Yield: 32 pieces.

Nutritional Values (per serving)

Calories:	47.8	Fiber:	.302 g
Carbohydrates:	5.15 g	Protein:	1.21 g
Cholesterol:	0 mg	Sodium:	17.2 mg
Fat:	2.53 g		

Mock Chocolate Cake

1 ¾ cups flour
⅓ cup carob powder
¾ cup sugar substitute
2 tablespoons instant dry milk
½ teaspoon cinnamon
¼ teaspoon salt substitute
2 teaspoons baking powder
1 cup lukewarm water
2 large eggs
⅓ cup polyunsaturated oil
1 ½ teaspoons vanilla extract

Preheat oven to 350° F. In a large bowl mix together
with a fork the flour, carob powder, sugar substitute,
dry milk, cinnamon, salt substitute and baking powder. In a separate small bowl, place the lukewarm
water, eggs, polyunsaturated oil and vanilla extract.
Use a wire whisk and briskly beat the ingredients
until well mixed and frothy. Add the frothy mixture
to the large bowl of mixed dry ingredients. Place the
batter in a 9" × 9" square nonstick cake pan. Bake 30
to 35 minutes. Cool on a wire rack. Cut in 2" squares.
Yield: 32 servings.

Nutritional Values (per serving)

Calories:	54.9	Fiber:	.651 g
Carbohydrates:	6.47 g	Protein:	1.24 g
Cholesterol:	13.4 mg	Sodium:	6.15 mg
Fat:	2.66 g		

Orange Pound Cake

½ cup diet margarine
⅓ cup sugar substitute
3 teaspoons orange extract
4 large eggs
1¾ cups flour
1½ teaspoons baking powder
¼ teaspoon salt substitute

Preheat oven to 350° F. In a large bowl, place the margarine, sugar substitute and orange extract. Beat until well blended. Add eggs to the blended mixture. Beat well. In a small bowl, mix together with a fork the flour, baking powder and salt substitute. Add to the mixture in the large bowl, a little at a time, beating well. Place the batter in a 9"×5" nonstick loaf pan. Bake for 1 hour. Remove to a wire rack and allow to cool completely. Cut cake ½" thick. Yield: 18 pieces.

Nutritional Values (per serving)

Calories:	82.9	Fiber:	.398 g
Carbohydrates:	9.61 g	Protein:	2.67 g
Cholesterol:	47.3 mg	Sodium:	36.8 mg
Fat:	3.68 g		

Chocolate Cake

1 cup flour
½ cup sugar substitute
3 tablespoons carob powder
1½ teaspoons baking powder
½ cup evaporated skim milk
2 tablespoons polyunsaturated oil
1 teaspoon vanilla extract
1 cup brown sugar substitute
½ cup carob powder
1¾ cups boiling water

Preheat oven to 350° F. Use a 9"×9" square nonstick cake pan. In the pan, place the flour, sugar substitute, 3 tablespoons carob powder, baking powder and evaporated skim milk. Mix well with a wooden spoon so as not to scratch the nonstick surface of your cake pan. When well blended, add the polyunsaturated oil and vanilla extract, and stir until well blended. In a small bowl, mix the 1 cup brown sugar and ½ cup carob powder together. Sprinkle the blended mixture over the batter in the cake pan. Pour the boiling water on top of the mixture. Do NOT stir. Bake for 40 minutes. Yield: 16 2"-square pieces.

Nutritional Values (per serving)

Calories:	54.3	Fiber:	.736 g
Carbohydrates:	7.95 g	Protein:	1.47 g
Cholesterol:	.287 mg	Sodium:	9.74 mg
Fat:	1.8 g		

Peach Upside-Down Cake

¾ cup packed brown sugar substitute
1 tablespoon polyunsaturated oil
2 teaspoons water
1 cup frozen sliced peaches, thawed and drained
1 cup fresh cranberries
¾ cup sugar substitute
¼ cup skim milk
¼ cup plain nonfat yogurt
3 tablespoons polyunsaturated oil
1 teaspoon vanilla extract
1¼ cups sifted cake flour
½ teaspoon baking powder
⅛ teaspoon salt substitute
2 egg whites

Preheat oven to 350° F. In a small saucepan, combine the brown sugar substitute, 1 tablespoon polyunsaturated oil and water. Stir well. Cook over medium heat until the brown sugar substitute dissolves. Stir occasionally. Pour the mixture into a 9"×9" square nonstick cake pan. Arrange the peach slices in the bottom of the pan. Place the cranberries over the peach slices. Set aside. In a small bowl, combine ¾ cup sugar substitute, skim milk, yogurt, 3 tablespoons polyunsaturated oil and vanilla extract. Stir well with a wire whisk.

In a large bowl, combine the sifted cake flour, baking powder and salt. Stir well with a fork. Add the ingredients from the small bowl to the large bowl, a little at a time. Beat until well blended. Set aside. Place the egg whites in a small bowl and beat until stiff peaks form. Fold the egg white mixture into the large bowl of mixed ingredients. Pour the batter on top of ingredients in the cake pan. Bake for 40 minutes. Immediately invert the cake onto a serving platter. Allow to cool. Yield: 32 ½" square × 2" thick pieces.

Nutritional Values (per serving)

Calories:	23.9	Fiber:	.259 g
Carbohydrates:	4.16 g	Protein:	.752 g
Cholesterol:	.069 mg	Sodium:	5.98 mg
Fat:	.176 g		

Almond Pound Cake

2/3 cup sugar substitute
2/3 cup Prune Purée (page 152)
1/4 cup diet margarine
1/2 teaspoon almond extract
1/2 teaspoon vanilla extract
2 egg whites
1 egg
1 3/4 cups flour
2 teaspoons baking powder
1/2 teaspoon ground allspice
1/8 teaspoon salt substitute
1/3 cup skim milk

Preheat oven to 350° F. In a large bowl, mix the sugar substitute, Prune Purée, margarine, almond extract, vanilla extract and the 2 egg whites. Beat well. Add the egg. Beat well. In another bowl, place the flour, baking powder, ground allspice and salt substitute. Stir with a fork to mix. Then begin adding the dry mixture to the mixture in the large bowl. Alternate this with the skim milk. Keep adding the ingredients until all are well blended. Pour the batter into an 8 1/2" × 4 1/2" loaf pan. Bake for 1 hour. Let cool to warm on a wire rack. Serve with the Lemon Sauce (below). Yield: 20 servings 1" thick × 4 1/2".

Lemon Sauce

1 cup apple cider
½ cup sugar substitute
1 tablespoon cornstarch
⅛ teaspoon salt substitute
1 teaspoon grated lemon rind
¼ cup fresh lemon juice

In a small saucepan, cook the apple cider, sugar substitute, cornstarch and salt substitute. Stir with a wire whisk until well blended. Bring mixture to a boil for 1 minute or until thickened. Be sure to stir constantly. Remove from heat. Add the grated lemon rind and lemon juice. Pour over each serving of pound cake. Serve immediately.

Nutritional Values (per serving)

Calories:	56.8	Fiber:	.358 g
Carbohydrates:	8.82 g	Protein:	1.95 g
Cholesterol:	10.7 mg	Sodium:	21.3 mg
Fat:	1.47 g		

Cranberry Banana Loaf Cake

2 cups flour
²⁄₃ cup firmly packed brown sugar substitute
¹⁄₃ cup sugar substitute
2 teaspoons baking powder
¹⁄₈ teaspoon salt substitute
2 cups mashed very ripe bananas
¹⁄₄ cup water
¹⁄₄ cup polyunsaturated oil
1 teaspoon vanilla extract
3 egg whites, lightly beaten
³⁄₄ cup chopped cranberries
¹⁄₄ cup chopped walnuts

Preheat oven to 350° F. In a large bowl, mix well the flour, brown sugar substitute, sugar substitute, baking powder and salt substitute. In a separate bowl, mix together the mashed bananas, water, polyunsaturated oil, vanilla, egg whites and chopped cranberries. Add the mixture, a little at a time, to the large bowl of dry ingredients. Mix very well. Pour the batter into a 9"×5" nonstick loaf pan. Sprinkle the chopped walnuts over the top. Bake for 65 minutes. Remove from the oven and place on a wire rack to cool. Yield: 32 ½" thick slices.

Nutritional Values (per piece)

Calories:	64.4	Fiber:	.659 g
Carbohydrates:	9.73 g	Protein:	1.28 g
Cholesterol:	0 mg	Sodium:	3.32 mg
Fat:	2.43 g		

Cranberry Loaf Cake

2 cups flour
2/3 cup firmly packed brown sugar substitute
1/3 cup sugar substitute
2 teaspoons baking powder
1/8 teaspoon salt substitute
1 3/4 teaspoons pumpkin pie spice
1 cup unsweetened canned pumpkin
1/4 cup water
1/4 cup polyunsaturated oil
1 1/2 teaspoons vanilla extract
3 egg whites, lightly beaten
3/4 cup chopped cranberries
1/4 cup chopped pecans

Preheat oven to 350° F. In a large bowl, mix well the flour, brown sugar substitute, sugar substitute, baking powder, salt substitute and pumpkin pie spice. In a separate bowl, mix together the unsweetened canned pumpkin, water, polyunstaurated oil, vanilla, egg whites and chopped cranberries. Add the mixture, a little at a time, to the large bowl of dry ingredients. Mix very well. Pour the batter into a 9"×5" nonstick loaf pan. Sprinkle the chopped pecans over the top. Bake for 65 minutes. Remove from the oven and place on a wire rack to cool. Yield: 32 1/2" thick slices.

Nutritional Values (per piece)

Calories:	56	Fiber:	.804 g
Carbohydrates:	7.22 g	Protein:	1.06 g
Cholesterol:	0 mg	Sodium:	.957 mg
Fat:	2.46 g		

Carrot Cake

2 ½ cups flour
1 cup sugar substitute
2 teaspoons baking soda
2 teaspoons ground cinnamon
2 8-ounce cans dietetic crushed pineapple, undrained
¼ cup skim milk
4 egg whites
2 teaspoons vanilla extract
2 cups grated carrots
½ cup golden raisins

Preheat oven to 325° F. In a large bowl, place the flour, sugar substitute, baking soda and cinnamon. Mix well. Add the canned pineapple and the juice, skim milk, egg whites and vanilla extract. Beat well. Fold in the carrots and raisins until well mixed. Use a 9" × 13" nonstick pan. Bake at 325° F for 35 minutes. Check with a wood toothpick. When the toothpick inserted into the middle of the cake comes out clean, the cake is done. Remove and set aside. Let the cake cool to room temperature. While cake is cooling, prepare the icing.

Icing

8 ounces nonfat cream cheese
1 cup nonfat ricotta cheese
½ cup powdered Isomalt®

Place all ingredients in a small bowl. Beat until smooth. Frost the top of the cake. Cake will be 2½" thick. Cut into 3" squares. Yield: 50 pieces.

Nutritional Values (per piece)

Calories:	35.9	Fiber:	.496 g
Carbohydrates:	8.02 g	Protein:	.829 g
Cholesterol:	.022 mg	Sodium:	52.9 mg
Fat:	.095 g		

Lemon Cheesecake

1 Graham Cracker Crust (page 134)
1 8-ounce package Philadelphia light cream cheese
2 cups cold milk
1 3-ounce package sugar-free instant lemon pudding
   mix
½ teaspoon grated lemon peel

Prepare graham cracker crust. Place in a 9"×9" pie pan. Set aside. In a large bowl, place the cream cheese. Beat well. Gradually add milk ½ cup at a time. Beat well. Add the lemon pudding mix. Beat well. Add the lemon peel and beat well. Continue beating until mixture is thick. Pour into the prepared graham cracker crust. Refrigerate for at least 3 hours or place in freezer until ready to serve. The cheesecake thaws quickly. Yield: 10 wedges.

Nutritional Values (per serving)

Calories:	121	Fiber:	.364 g
Carbohydrates:	17.9 g	Protein:	4.73 g
Cholesterol:	1.84 mg	Sodium:	189 mg
Fat:	3.54 g		

Crunchy Chocolate Cupcakes

1½ cups flour
¾ cup wheat germ
¼ cup sugar substitute
1 tablespoon baking powder
1 cup skim milk
¼ cup diet margarine, melted
1 egg
1 cup carob chips

Preheat oven to 400° F. Place paper cups in muffin tins and set aside. In a large bowl, mix the flour, wheat germ, sugar substitute and baking powder together with a fork. Set aside. In a small bowl, mix together the skim milk, diet margarine and egg. Beat well. Slowly add the mixture from the small bowl to the large bowl. Beat well. Add carob chips and mix well. Place batter in cupcake paper cups in muffin tins. Fill the cups half full. Bake 20 to 25 minutes. Yield: 24 1½" diameter × 2" deep cupcakes.

Nutritional Values (per serving)

Calories:	96.7	Fiber:	.721 g
Carbohydrates:	13.5 g	Protein:	3.3 g
Cholesterol:	.94 mg	Sodium:	14.6 mg
Fat:	3.4 g		

Date Cupcakes

2 cups flour
1 teaspoon baking powder
1 teaspoon baking soda
1/4 teaspoon salt substitute
2 teaspoons grated orange rind
1/2 cup sugar substitute
1 medium-sized orange, peeled and sectioned
1/2 cup diet margarine
1/2 cup chopped dates
1/2 cup orange juice
1 egg

Preheat oven to 400° F. Place the flour, baking powder, baking soda, salt substitute, grated orange rind and sugar substitute in a large bowl. Mix well. In a blender, place the orange sections, diet margarine, dates, orange juice and egg. Blend at medium speed until ingredients are well blended but lumpy. Add the blended ingredients to the mixture in the bowl. You may use paper cupcake cups if you so desire. Spoon the batter into the paper cupcake holders or directly into your muffin tin. Fill half full. Bake in the oven for 15 minutes. Yield: 24 cupcakes, 2" diameter × 1 1/2" deep.

Nutritional Values (per piece)

Calories:	72.1	Fiber:	.712 g
Carbohydrates:	11.9 g	Protein:	1.51 g
Cholesterol:	8.88 mg	Sodium:	19.8 mg
Fat:	2.17 g		

Cookies

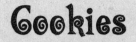

Banana Cookies

1 cup sugar substitute
½ cup diet margarine
⅓ cup mashed ripe banana
1 teaspoon vanilla extract
1 egg
2¼ cups flour
1 teaspoon baking soda
⅛ teaspoon ground nutmeg
1½ cups low fat granola

Preheat oven to 325° F. In a large bowl, cream the sugar substitute and diet margarine until fluffy. Add the mashed banana, vanilla extract and the egg. Beat well. In a small bowl place the flour, baking soda and nutmeg. Mix well with a fork. Add the dry mixture to the creamed mixture in the large bowl. Mix well. Drop by teaspoons onto a nonstick cookie sheet. Bake for 10 to 12 minutes. Remove cookies immediately from the cookie sheet to a wire rack to cool. Cookies will be 1" diameter. Yield: 72 cookies.

Nutritional Values (per piece)

Calories:	29.2	Fiber:	.275 g
Carbohydrates:	4.82 g	Protein:	.698 g
Cholesterol:	2.96 mg	Sodium:	10.3 mg
Fat:	.851 g		

Carob Chip Cookies

2 1/4 cups flour
1 teaspoon baking soda
1/4 teaspoon salt substitute
1/2 cup sugar substitute
3/4 cup brown sugar substitute
1/2 cup diet margarine
2 large eggs
1 teaspoon vanilla extract
2 1/2 cups carob chips

Preheat oven to 375° F. In a large bowl, mix together the flour, baking soda, salt substitute, sugar substitute and brown sugar substitute. Add the margarine and blend well. Add the eggs and vanilla extract. Beat well. Add the carob chips and mix well. Drop by 1" diameter spoonfuls onto an ungreased baking sheet. Bake 7 to 10 minutes. Yield: 72 cookies.

Nutritional Values (per piece)

Calories:	59	Fiber:	1.28 g
Carbohydrates:	7.33 g	Protein:	1.76 g
Cholesterol:	6.55 mg	Sodium:	7.38 mg
Fat:	2.52 g		

Oatmeal Cookies

1 cup polyunsaturated oil
¾ cup granulated sugar substitute
1 cup firmly packed brown sugar substitute
2 large eggs
1 teaspoon vanilla extract
2 cups flour
1 teaspoon baking soda
½ teaspoon baking powder
½ teaspoon salt substitute
2 cups uncooked oatmeal
1 cup shredded coconut

Preheat oven to 350° F. Place the oil, granulated sugar substitute and imitation brown sugar in a bowl. Beat well. Add eggs and vanilla extract. Mix well. Add the flour, baking soda, baking powder and salt substitute to the beaten mixture a little at a time. Mix well with each addition of ingredients. Add the oats and coconut. Mix well. Shape into 1" diameter balls. Place on a cookie sheet. With a fork, flatten each ball, leaving the fork prong imprints in the flattened ball. Place in the oven and bake 5 to 7 minutes. Yield: 84 cookies.

Nutritional Values (per piece)

Calories:	45.8	Fiber:	3.52 g
Carbohydrates:	3.29 g	Protein:	.665 g
Cholesterol:	5.07 mg	Sodium:	18 mg
Fat:	3.4 g		

Carob and Coconut Macaroons

1 cup carob chips
2 large egg whites
¼ teaspoon cream of tartar
⅓ cup sugar substitute
1 teaspoon vanilla extract
2½ cups grated coconut

Preheat oven to 375° F. Place the carob chips in the top of a double boiler. Melt carob chips. While carob chips are melting, place the egg whites and cream of tartar in a large bowl. Beat the egg whites and cream of tartar until it holds stiff peaks. Fold in the melted carob chips, sugar substitute, and vanilla extract. Add the grated coconut. Place by teaspoonfuls on a nonstick cookie sheet. Bake for 20 minutes. Remove from oven and place on a wire rack to cool. Yield: 40 1" diameter macaroons.

Nutritional Values (per piece)

Calories:	56.1	Fiber:	.838 g
Carbohydrates:	3.56 g	Protein:	1.28 g
Cholesterol:	11 mg	Sodium:	4.97 mg
Fat:	4.33 g		

Cherry Coconut Macaroons

2 large egg whites
¼ teaspoon cream of tartar
⅓ cup sugar substitute
1 teaspoon almond extract
2¼ cups grated coconut

Preheat oven to 375° F. Place the egg whites and cream of tartar in a large bowl. Beat until stiff peaks form. Continue beating, adding the sugar substitute. Fold in the almond extract. Then fold in the grated coconut. Mixture will be stiff. Drop by teaspoonsful onto a nonstick cookie sheet. Bake 20 minutes. Remove macaroons to a wire rack to cool. Cookies will be 1" in diameter. Yield: 35 pieces.

Nutritional Values (per piece)

Calories:	34.1	Fiber:	.826 g
Carbohydrates:	1.26 g	Protein:	.546 g
Cholesterol:	0 mg	Sodium:	5 mg
Fat:	3.23 g		

Lemon Biscotti

3 1/2 cups flour
1 tablespoon baking powder
1/2 cup margarine
1/2 cup sugar substitute
5 eggs
2 tablespoons freshly grated lemon peel
1 teaspoon vanilla extract
1 cup pine nuts
3/4 cup pistachio nuts
1 egg white, lightly beaten
3/4 teaspoon powdered Isomalt®

In a large bowl, combine the flour and baking powder. In another large bowl, combine the margarine and sugar substitute. Beat until fluffy and light in color. Add the 5 eggs, lemon peel and vanilla extract. Beat until mixture is smooth and thick. Add the flour gradually. Mix well after each addition. Add the pine nuts and the pistachio nuts. Blend well. Gather the dough into a ball. Divide the dough into 3 equal parts. Wrap each part in plastic wrap. Refrigerate for 5 hours.

Preheat the oven to 350° F. Use a nonstick baking sheet or lightly grease a baking sheet with low-calorie cooking spray.

Remove the dough from the refrigerator. Transfer each section to a lightly floured surface. Shape each portion into a large log. Place 2 of the logs on 1 sheet about 5 inches apart. Place the remaining log on another cooking sheet. Brush each log with the egg white. Sprinkle with ¼ teaspoon powdered Isomalt® on each log.

Place the logs in the oven. Bake 30 to 35 minutes or until the dough has flattened somewhat and the top is slightly cracked. Remove from the oven. Using a large metal spatula, loosen the dough from the sheet. Leave on the sheet for 10 minutes. Carefully transfer the logs, one at a time, to a cutting board.

With a large knife, slice each log into diagonal slices that are 3" long by ¼" thick. Return the sliced biscotti to the baking sheets. Bake for 10 to 15 minutes, turning twice, until the biscotti are dry and lightly toasted. Remove from oven and cool on racks. Yield: 60 pieces.

Nutritional Values (per piece)

Calories:	69.3	Fiber:	.836 g
Carbohydrates:	6.88 g	Protein:	2.03 g
Cholesterol:	13.1 mg	Sodium:	15.4 mg
Fat:	4.2 g		

Lemon Squares

1 cup margarine
½ cup sugar substitute
½ teaspoon salt substitute
1 egg
1 egg yolk
2 tablespoons fresh lemon juice
1 teaspoon vanilla extract
4 cups floor

Combine the margarine, sugar substitute and salt substitute together in a large bowl. Beat until light and fluffy. Add the egg, the egg yolk, lemon juice and vanilla extract. Beat until well blended. Then gradually add the flour. Beat until mixed.

Remove the dough from the bowl and form into 2 large balls. Wrap each large ball in plastic wrap. Place the wrapped balls in the refrigerator for 4 hours.

Preheat oven to 350° F. Use a greased baking sheet or a baking sheet with a nonstick surface.

Remove the dough from the refrigerator. On a lightly floured surface roll out each ball to ⅛ inch thickness. Using a sharp knife cut into 1" squares or use cookie cutters of this size. Place each cookie on the baking sheet 1" apart. Bake for 10 minutes. The edges should be a light brown. Remove from oven and place on racks to cool. Yield: 80 cookies.

Nutritional Values (per piece)

Calories:	33.4	Fiber:	.206 g
Carbohydrates:	4.82 g	Protein:	.719 g
Cholesterol:	1.96 mg	Sodium:	10.7 mg
Fat:	1.21 g		

Vanilla Drops

1 cup margarine
½ cup powdered Isomalt®
1 teaspoon vanilla extract
2 cups flour

In a large bowl, cream the margarine until light and fluffy. Add the powdered Isomalt® and vanilla extract. Beat well. Add the flour a little at a time. Mix well. Cover the bowl and place in the refrigerator for 30 minutes.

Preheat the oven to 375° F. Remove the dough from the refrigerator. Shape into 1" balls. Place 1" apart on an ungreased baking sheet. Bake 12 minutes. Cookies will be a light golden color. Place the cookies on a cooling rack.

While cookies are in the oven, powder ¼ cup Isomalt®. When cookies are on the cooling rack, dust each cookie with the powdered Isomalt®. Let cool. Yield: 60 cookies.

Nutritional Values (per piece)

Calories:	28.4	Fiber:	.136 g
Carbohydrates:	3.2 g	Protein:	.449 g
Cholesterol:	0 mg	Sodium:	13.4 mg
Fat:	1.51 g		

Peanut Butter Cookies

2 cups smooth dietetic peanut butter
1 cup sugar substitute
2 eggs
60 carob chips

Preheat the oven to 350° F. In a bowl, combine the peanut butter, sugar substitute and eggs. Blend thoroughly. Flour your hands and form the mixture into 2" diameter balls. Place the balls on an ungreased baking sheet. Make sure there are at least 2 inches between the balls. The cookies need plenty of room to spread. Then place a carob chip in the center of each cookie. Place in the oven and bake for 12 minutes. Remove from the oven and place on a cooling rack. Yield: 60 cookies.

Nutritional Values (per piece)

Calories:	53.1	Fiber:	.563 g
Carbohydrates:	1.97 g	Protein:	2.26 g
Cholesterol:	6.25 mg	Sodium:	2.36 mg
Fat:	4.43 g		

Heavenly Puffs

1 cup margarine
1 cup sugar substitute
2 eggs
2 ¾ cups flour
2 teaspoons cream of tartar
1 teaspoon baking soda
¼ teaspoon salt substitute
2 teaspoons ground cinnamon
¼ teaspoon sugar substitute

Place the margarine, 1 cup sugar substitute and eggs in a large bowl. Beat well. Mixture will be light and fluffy.

In a medium-sized bowl combine the flour, cream of tartar, baking soda and salt substitute. Mix well. Add this mixture to the light and fluffy mixture in the large bowl. Blend well. Cover the large bowl and place in the refrigerator for an hour.

Remove bowl from refrigerator. Preheat the oven to 375° F. In a small bowl, mix the cinnamon plus ¼ teaspoon sugar substitute. Mix well. Shape the dough in the large bowl into balls 2" in diameter. Roll in the cinnamon and sugar mixture. Place the balls 3" apart on an ungreased baking sheet. Bake the cookies 12 to 15 minutes (until golden brown). Yield: 35 cookies.

Nutritional Values (per piece)

Calories:	102	Fiber:	.743 g
Carbohydrates:	16 g	Protein:	2.51 g
Cholesterol:	12.2 mg	Sodium:	62.9 mg
Fat:	3.01 g		

Pies

Pie Crust

1 cup flour
1 teaspoon sugar substitute
¼ teaspoon salt substitute
3 tablespoons vegetable shortening
3 tablespoons ice water

In a bowl, combine the flour, sugar substitute and salt substitute. Add the vegetable shortening and cut with 2 knives or pastry cutter. Add the ice water and knead until well mixed. If needed, more ice water can be added. Place on a floured board. Roll out to desired thickness. Yield: 1 pie crust (10 slices).

Nutritional Values (per slice)

Calories:	68.2	Fiber:	.409 g
Carbohydrates:	9.54 g	Protein:	1.29 g
Cholesterol:	0 mg	Sodium:	.25 mg
Fat:	2.69 g		

Graham Cracker Crust

1 cup finely crushed graham crackers
¼ cup melted diet margarine

Preheat oven to 350° F. Combine the crushed graham crackers and melted diet margarine in a bowl. Mix well. Press into the bottom and on the sides of a 9" pie pan. Bake 8 to 10 minutes. Yield: 1 pie crust (10 slices).

Nutritional Values (per slice)

Calories:	70.4	Fiber:	.324 g
Carbohydrates:	9.24 g	Protein:	.856 g
Cholesterol:	0 mg	Sodium:	92.6 mg
Fat:	3.41 g		

Pumpkin Pie

1 Pie Crust (page 133)
1 large can pumpkin
1 cup evaporated milk
1 teaspoon pumpkin pie spice
1 teaspoon vanilla extract
3 egg yolks
10 teaspoons diet frozen whipped topping

Preheat oven to 350° F. Prepare pie crust. Place rolled
out crust in the bottom of a 9" pie pan. Flute edges of
crust. In a large bowl, place the pumpkin, evaporated
milk, pumpkin pie spice, vanilla extract and egg yolks.
Beat well with a wooden spoon. Continue beating
until well mixed. Then pour into pie shell. Sprinkle
top with nutmeg. Bake 40 to 45 minutes. Place on a
wire rack to cool. Then refrigerate. Cut into 10 wedges.
Place 1 teaspoon of diet frozen whipped topping on
each piece just before serving. Yield: 10 pieces.

Nutritional Values (per serving)

Calories:	58.1	Fiber:	1.27 g
Carbohydrates:	7.03 g	Protein:	3.29 g
Cholesterol:	64.8 mg	Sodium:	34.1 mg
Fat:	2.11 g		

Apple Pie

2 Pie Crusts (page 133)
8 cooking apples, peeled, cored and sliced
1 tablespoon lemon juice
2 tablespoons flour
1 teaspoon cinnamon
1/2 teaspoon nutmeg
1/8 teaspoon ginger

Preheat oven to 350° F. In a large bowl place the peeled, cored and sliced apples. Add lemon juice, flour, cinnamon, nutmeg and ginger. Mix well. Roll out the pie crust. Place the pie crust in a 9" pie pan. Add the apple mixture. Roll out another pie crust and place on top of apple mixture. Slice to release steam. Flute edges. Bake 40 minutes. Can be served warm or when cooled. Yield: 10 pieces.

Nutritional Values (per serving)

Calories:	71.2	Fiber:	2.23 g
Carbohydrates:	18.2 g	Protein:	.377 g
Cholesterol:	0 mg	Sodium:	.047 mg
Fat:	.415 g		

Peach Pie

2 Pie Crusts (page 133)
5 cups sliced fresh peaches
¼ cup flour
1 teaspoon lemon juice
1 teaspoon cinnamon
1 teaspoon allspice
10 teaspoons diet frozen whipped topping

Preheat oven to 425° F. In a bowl, mix together the peaches, flour, lemon juice, cinnamon and allspice. Place a rolled out pie crust in a 9" pie pan. Roll out a second piece for the top of the pie. Place the peach mixture in the pie pan on top of the crust. Place the second piece of rolled out pie crust on top of peach mixture. Cut a design for steam to be released. Flute the edges. Bake at 425° F for 15 minutes. Then reduce the heat to 350° F, and continue to bake for 25 minutes. Cool. Cut into 10 2" wedges. Place 1 teaspoon of diet frozen whipped topping on each wedge. Serve immediately. Yield: 10 pieces.

Nutritional Values (per serving)

Calories:	52	Fiber:	1.63 g
Carbohydrates:	12.2 g	Protein:	.935 g
Cholesterol:	0 mg	Sodium:	.384 mg
Fat:	.425 g		

Avocado Pie

Pie crust

¾ cup fat-free graham cracker crumbs
¾ teaspoon sugar substitute
4 egg whites

Place graham cracker crumbs, sugar substitute and egg whites in a blender. Process until the mixture is moist and crumbly. Place mixture in an 8" pie pan. Press mixture into the bottom of the pan and up the sides.

Filling

¼ cup hot water
1 package Knox gelatin
2 medium-sized avocados
1 can condensed milk
2 tablespoons lemon juice
1 cup diet whipped topping

In a small bowl, place the hot water and Knox gelatin. Set aside. Place the avocados, condensed milk, lemon juice and Knox gelatin mixture in a blender. Blend until well mixed. Pour into pie crust. Spread the dairy topping over the top. Refrigerate for 2 hours. Yield: 8 wedges.

Nutritional Values (per serving)

Calories:	238	Fiber:	2.08 g
Carbohydrates:	27 g	Protein:	4.91 g
Cholesterol:	13 mg	Sodium:	57.8 mg
Fat:	13.4 g		

Pineapple Pie

1 Graham Cracker Crust (page 134)
1 package (1 ounce) sugar-free instant vanilla pudding
   mix
1 cup diet sour cream
1 cup dietetic canned crushed pineapple, drained
½ teaspoon sugar substitute

Prepare graham cracker crust. Place crust in a 9" pie
pan. In a bowl, combine the pudding mix and sour
cream. Beat well until completely blended. Add the
pineapple. Stir well. Add the sugar substitute. Stir
until well blended. Pour into the prepared graham
cracker crust. Refrigerate for 4 hours before serving.
Yield: 10 pieces.

Nutritional Values (per serving)

Calories:	92.8	Fiber:	.512 g
Carbohydrates:	12.4 g	Protein:	1.69 g
Cholesterol:	9.44 mg	Sodium:	87.7 mg
Fat:	4.21 g		

Hodge Podge

Raspberry Crunch

½ cup fresh raspberries, crushed
1 cup margarine
1 cup sugar substitute
2 teaspoons vanilla extract
2 egg yolks
2 ½ cups sifted flour
1 cup chopped pecans

Place the raspberries in a blender. Blend at low speed until raspberries are crushed but not liquid. Place the margarine, sugar substitute, vanilla and egg yolks in a bowl. Beat at high speed until light and fluffy. Gradually stir in the flour as you continue to beat. When completely blended, shape into a ball and place in a plastic bag or plastic wrap. Put in the refrigerator and leave for 4 hours.

Preheat the oven to 300° F. Remove the dough from the refrigerator. Shape the dough into 1" balls. Place the balls on a cookie sheet 1 ½" apart. Using a wooden spoon, make an indentation in the center of each cookie. Fill each cookie with 1 teaspoon of fresh, crushed raspberries. Bake the cookies for 20 minutes. Remove to cooling racks. Yield: 48 cookies.

Nutritional Values (per piece)

Calories:	55.9	Fiber:	.339 g
Carbohydrates:	5.24 g	Protein:	1.06 g
Cholesterol:	8.88 mg	Sodium:	20 mg
Fat:	3.45 g		

Sweet Snack

3 cups presweetened carob chips
1 cup banana chips
1 cup raisins
1 cup chopped English walnuts
1 cup chopped peanuts

Place the presweetened carob chips in the top of a double boiler and melt. Add the banana chips, raisins, English walnuts and peanuts. Mix well. Drop by 1" balls onto waxed paper. Place in the refrigerator to cool. Yield: 60 1" snacks.

Nutritional Values (per piece)

Calories:	60.2	Fiber:	.461 mg
Carbohydrates:	5.78 g	Protein:	1.54 g
Cholesterol:	.302 mg	Sodium:	.728 mg
Fat:	3.81 g		

Trail Mix

20 unsalted low-fat saltine crackers
1 cup raisins
1 cup peanuts
2 cups presweetened carob chips

In a medium-sized bowl, crumble the saltine crackers into bite-sized pieces. Add the raisins, peanuts and carob chips. Mix well. Place in the refrigerator. Measure ½ cup each and place in plastic sandwich-sized bags. Yield: 65 servings.

Nutritional Values (per serving)

Calories:	30.6	Fiber:	.274 g
Carbohydrates:	3.83 g	Protein:	.876 g
Cholesterol:	.07 mg	Sodium:	10.2 mg
Fat:	1.5 g		

Spice Delight

4 cups flour
1 teaspoon ground cinnamon
1 teaspoon ground nutmeg
½ teaspoon ground ginger
¼ teaspoon ground cloves
1½ cups margarine
½ cup sugar substitute
1 egg
1 teaspoon vanilla extract

In a large bowl, combine the flour, cinnamon, nutmeg, ginger, and cloves. In another large bowl, beat the margarine and sugar substitute together until light and fluffy. Add the egg and the vanilla extract. Beat until well blended. Then with the mixer on low speed, gradually add the flour and spice mixture. Mix until well blended.

Separate the dough into 3 equal parts. Flatten each piece to 1" thick. Wrap in plastic wrap and refrigerate for 1 hour.

Preheat oven to 375° F. Remove the dough from the refrigerator. On a lightly floured surface, roll out each of the 3 sections, 1 section at a time, to ¼" thick. Use a cookie cutter for fun shapes or a sharp knife and cut into 1" squares. Place the cookies 1" apart on an ungreased baking sheet. Bake for 10 minutes or until the edges are lightly browned. Place cookies on a rack to cool. Yield: 80 cookies.

Nutritional Values (per piece)

Calories:	38.5	Fiber:	.23 g
Carbohydrates:	4.84 g	Protein:	.728 g
Cholesterol:	1.96 mg	Sodium:	15.7 mg
Fat:	1.77 g		

Chocolate Bars

1 cup firmly packed brown sugar substitute
1 cup diet margarine
1 egg yolk
1 teaspoon vanilla extract
2 cups flour
1/8 teaspoon salt substitute
2 cups melted carob
1 cup finely chopped walnuts

Preheat oven to 350°F. In a large mixing bowl, cream the brown sugar substitute and the diet margarine together. Add the egg yolk, vanilla extract, flour and salt substitute. Mix well. Spread mixture in a 9" × 13" nonstick pan. Bake 20 to 25 minutes. While bars are baking, melt carob in the top of a double boiler. When bars are removed from the oven, pour the melted carob over the bars. Then sprinkle the chopped walnuts on top of the carob bars. Let cool completely. Cut into 2" long × 1" wide bars. Bars will be 1" thick. Yield: 72 bars.

Nutritional Values (per piece)

Calories:	54.2	Fiber:	.114 g
Carbohydrates:	6.12 g	Protein:	1.35 g
Cholesterol:	3.46 mg	Sodium:	11.3 mg
Fat:	2.72 g		

Maple Bars

1 cup packed brown sugar substitute
1/3 cup diet margarine
1 1/2 teaspoons maple extract
1 teaspoon vanilla extract
1 egg
1 egg white
2 cups flour
3/4 teaspoon baking soda
1/2 teaspoon ground cinnamon
1/4 teaspoon ground allspice

Preheat oven to 325° F. In a small bowl, combine the brown sugar substitute and diet margarine. Beat until fluffy. Add the maple extract, vanilla extract, egg and egg white. Beat very well. In a large bowl, combine the flour, baking soda, cinnamon and allspice. Mix together with a fork. Add the ingredients from the small bowl to the large bowl, a little at a time. Stir well. Drop by teaspoons onto a nonstick cooking sheet. Shape into bars. Place in the oven and bake 8 to 10 minutes. Cookies will be 1" long × 1/4" wide × 1/4" deep. Yield: 72 bars.

Nutritional Values (per piece)

Calories:	17.3	Fiber:	.114 g
Carbohydrates:	2.66 g	Protein:	.45 g
Cholesterol:	2.96 mg	Sodium:	17.8 mg
Fat:	.512 g		

Brownies

1 cup sugar substitute
¼ cup polyunsaturated oil
¼ cup plain nonfat yogurt
1 teaspoon vanilla extract
3 egg whites
½ cup flour
½ cup powdered carob
¼ teaspoon baking powder
⅛ teaspoon salt substitute
¼ cup carob chips

Preheat oven to 375° F. In a large bowl, combine the sugar substitute, oil, yogurt, vanilla extract and egg whites. Mix well. Set aside. In another bowl combine the flour, powdered carob, baking powder and salt substitute. Mix well. Add this mixture to the mixture in the large bowl. Mix until well moistened. Place the mixture in a 9" square nonstick cake pan. Bake for 25 minutes. Remove from the oven and sprinkle the top with ¼ cup carob chips. Let stand until the carob chips begin to melt. Spread over the top of the brownies with a spatula. Cool. Yield: 36 1" square brownies.

Nutritional Values (per piece)

Calories:	38.2	Fiber:	.626 g
Carbohydrates:	4.03 g	Protein:	.852 g
Cholesterol:	.292 mg	Sodium:	4.32 mg
Fat:	2.09 g		

Fruit Crêpes

2 eggs, beaten
1 cup whole milk
1 cup flour
4 sliced, cored and peeled apples
¼ teaspoon cinnamon
1 teaspoon polyunsaturated oil

Place the eggs in a medium-sized bowl and beat well. Add the milk and flour. Mix well. Cover the bowl and allow to stand at room temperature for 30 minutes. Prepare the apples by slicing, coring and peeling. Add cinnamon to prepared apples. Stir well to coat the sliced apples. Heat and add 1 teaspoon polyunsaturated oil to a 6" frying pan (or use a nonstick crêpe pan). Pour batter to cover bottom of pan. When light brown, turn and brown the other side. Remove from heat. Add 1 tablespoon prepared apples to half of the cooked crêpe. Fold top over the apples and place on serving plate. Yield: 12 crêpes.

Nutritional Values (per serving)

Calories:	58.3	Fiber:	.907 g
Carbohydrates:	8.14 g	Protein:	2.32 g
Cholesterol:	56 mg	Sodium:	25.8 mg
Fat:	2.1 g		

Prune Purée

¼ cup diet maple syrup
2 tablespoons sugar substitute
1 12-ounce package whole, pitted prunes
⅔ cup water

In a food blender, place the diet maple syrup, sugar substitute and the prunes. Blend well. Slowly add the water. Blend until mixture is smooth. Purée can be used in recipes noted in this cookbook or use on toast for a special treat. Yield: 2 cups.

Nutritional Values (2 cups)

Calories:	454	Fiber:	15.7 g
Carbohydrates:	119 g	Protein:	4.45 g
Cholesterol:	0 mg	Sodium:	63.5 mg
Fat:	.885 g		

Chocolate Soufflé

5 tablespoons sugar substitute
½ cup Prune Purée (page 152)
2 ounces sweetened carob, grated
6 egg whites
¼ teaspoon cream of tartar
⅛ teaspoon salt substitute

Coat a 1½ quart soufflé pan with diet cooking spray.
Sprinkle with 1 tablespoon sugar substitute and set
aside. Preheat oven to 350° F. In a medium bowl, combine 2 tablespoons sugar substitute, Prune Purée and
grated carob. Set aside. In another bowl, beat the egg
whites, cream of tartar and salt substitute until soft
peaks form. Gradually add the remaining 2 tablespoons sugar substitute and beat until stiff peaks
form. Fold the egg white mixture into the Prune Purée mixture. Spoon the mixture into the soufflé pan.
Place the soufflé pan in a 9"×9" square baking pan.
Add hot water to the pan to 1" depth. Gently place in
the preheated oven and bake for 55 minutes. If you
desire, sprinkle the top with ⅛ teaspoon sugar substitute. Serve immediately. Yield: 12 2-ounce servings.

Nutritional Values (per serving)

Calories:	40.2	Fiber:	1.54 g
Carbohydrates:	10.3 g	Protein:	.333 g
Cholesterol:	0 mg	Sodium:	5.26 mg
Fat:	.059 g		

Custard Tarts

1 cup flour
⅓ cup unsalted margarine
4 tablespoons unsweetened apple juice
¾ cup sugar-free applesauce
½ cup whole milk
2 eggs
½ teaspoon cinnamon
1 apple, sliced and cored

Preheat oven to 425° F. In a medium-sized bowl, combine the flour and margarine. Add enough fruit juice to form a soft dough. Knead well. Pinch off small pieces and press into nonstick tart pans or small muffin tin wells. Set aside. In a blender, place the applesauce, milk, eggs and cinnamon. Blend well. Fill each tart ¾ full. Sprinkle tops with cinnamon. Bake at 425° F for 10 minutes. Then reduce heat to 350° F. Continue baking another 20 to 25 minutes. Place on wire rack to cool. Refrigerate 1 hour. When ready to serve, place one apple slice on top of each tart. Yield: 20 tarts.

Nutritional Values (per serving)

Calories:	56.9	Fiber:	.355 g
Carbohydrates:	7.63 g	Protein:	1.52 g
Cholesterol:	22.1 mg	Sodium:	23.6 mg
Fat:	2.27 g		

Peach Tarts

1 cup flour
⅓ cup diet margarine
4 tablespoons unsweetened apple juice
2¼ cups chopped fresh peaches
3 tablespoons cornstarch

Preheat oven to 375° F. In a medium-sized bowl, mix together the flour, diet margarine and unsweetened apple juice. Knead well. Break off small pieces and press into nonstick tart pans or small muffin tin wells. Place the peaches and cornstarch in a blender and blend well. Then pour into the top of a double boiler. Heat over medium heat, stirring constantly until mixture thickens. Remove from heat. Fill each tart half full. Bake for 20 to 25 minutes. Place on wire rack to cool. Sprinkle cooled tarts with cinnamon or nutmeg if you desire. Yield: 20 tarts.

Nutritional Values (per serving)

Calories:	54.4	Fiber:	.574 g
Carbohydrates:	9.45 g	Protein:	.819 g
Cholesterol:	0 mg	Sodium:	14.4 mg
Fat:	1.56 g		

Pumpkin Tarts

1 Pie Crust (page 133)
1 cup unsweetened canned pumpkin
1 cup whole milk
½ cup sugar substitute
¾ teaspoon vanilla extract
½ teaspoon pumpkin pie spice
¼ teaspoon butter-flavored extract
2 eggs, beaten lightly
2 egg whites, beaten lightly
⅓ cup nondairy whipped topping

Preheat oven to 350° F. Make the pie crust. Before rolling out, set aside. In a large bowl, combine the above ingredients. Mix very well. Set aside. Roll out the pie crust. Place in a 10" round nonstick tart pan. Prick the bottom of the crust with a fork in several places. Place the pumpkin mixture in the crust. Bake for 40 minutes. The filling will be almost set. Remove from oven. Cool at least 30 to 40 minutes. Spread the nondairy topping on the tart. Cut into wedges 1" across. Serve immediately. Yield: 40 tarts.

Nutritional Values (per serving)

Calories:	12.3	Fiber:	.172 g
Carbohydrates:	.973 g	Protein:	.75 g
Cholesterol:	11.5 g	Sodium:	9.11 mg
Fat:	.63 g		

Frozen Fruit

2 cans dietetic crushed pineapple, undrained
1 can dietetic cherry pie filling
1 can evaporated skim milk
1 8-ounce carton diet frozen whipped topping (thawed)
36 green or red maraschino cherries

In a large bowl, mix the dietetic crushed pineapple, dietetic cherry pie filling and evaporated skim milk. Fold in the diet frozen whipped topping. Blend well. Pour mixture into a 13" × 9" nonstick pan. Cover and place in the freezer at least 2 hours or until thoroughly frozen. When ready to serve, cut and place 1 maraschino cherry on each piece. Cut pieces 2" × 2" square. Yield: 36 pieces.

Nutritional Values (per piece)

Calories:	41	Fiber:	.254 g
Carbohydrates:	6.01 g	Protein:	.79 g
Cholesterol:	.283 mg	Sodium:	11.5 mg
Fat:	1.75 g		

Haupia
(Hawaiian Sweet Treat)

3 packages Knox gelatin
½ cup water
1 can coconut milk
⅔ cup sugar substitute
1 cup skim milk

Combine the 3 packages of Knox gelatin and ½ cup water. Set aside. In a heavy pot, combine the coconut milk and sugar substitute. Heat until the sugar substitute dissolves. Do not boil. Add the gelatin mixture. Stir well. Remove from heat. Add the skim milk. Mix well. Allow mixture to cool. Stir the mixture again as it begins to gel. Then pour into an 8"×8" square pan. Refrigerate. Cut into 2" squares. Mixture will be 2" square×1" thick. Yield: 80 pieces.

Nutritional Values (per piece)

Calories:	7.51	Fiber:	.032 g
Carbohydrates:	.228 g	Protein:	.387 g
Cholesterol:	.055 mg	Sodium:	2.46 mg
Fat:	.607 g		

Maple Pudding

1 package sugar-free maple pudding and pie
  filling mix
1 8-ounce carton plain low-fat yogurt
1 8-ounce carton vanilla low-fat yogurt
1 cup chopped English walnuts
½ cup diet frozen whipped topping (thawed)

In a large bowl, place the maple pudding mix, plain low-fat yogurt, vanilla low-fat yogurt and chopped English walnuts. Mix well. Fold in the thawed frozen whipped topping. Spoon ½ cup each into serving bowls. Refrigerate 3 hours before serving. If desired, sprinkle top with a dash of ground cinnamon. Yield: 12 servings.

Nutritional Values (per serving)

Calories:	100	Fiber:	.456 g
Carbohydrates:	6.15 g	Protein:	3.98 g
Cholesterol:	1.05 mg	Sodium:	41.7 mg
Fat:	7.15 g		

Cherry Scones

¾ cup dried cherries
¼ cup boiling water
1¾ cups flour
½ cup sugar substitute
¼ cup yellow cornmeal
2 teaspoons baking powder
⅛ teaspoon salt substitute
2 tablespoons diet margarine
⅓ cup plain nonfat yogurt
¼ cup evaporated skim milk
1 teaspoon vanilla extract
½ teaspoon imitation butter extract
1 egg white, beaten lightly
3 teaspoons sugar substitute

Preheat oven to 425° F. In a bowl, place the cherries and the boiling water. Set aside. In a large bowl, mix the flour, ½ cup sugar substitute, cornmeal, baking powder and salt substitute. Cut in the diet margarine with two knives or a pastry blender. Mixture will be coarse. Drain the water off the softened cherries. Blend in the bowl with the cherries the yogurt, skim milk and extracts. Add the blended ingredients, a little at a time, to the dry ingredients mixed in the large bowl. Stir just until the dry ingredients are moist. The dough will be sticky. Place the sticky dough in an 8" × 8" square nonstick cake pan. Brush the beaten egg white over the top of the dough. Sprinkle the top of the egg whites with the 3 teaspoons sugar substitute. Bake in the oven for 20 minutes. Remove from oven. Can be served warm or when cooled. Yield: 16 scones.

Nutritional Values (per piece)

Calories:	110	Fiber:	1.05 g
Carbohydrates:	21.1 g	Protein:	2.75 g
Cholesterol:	.56 mg	Sodium:	21.8 mg
Fat:	2.73 g		

Bread Pudding

2 cups low-fat milk
1 cup egg substitute
¾ cup Prune Purée (page 152)
¾ cup sugar substitute
½ cup evaporated skim milk
2 tablespoons diet margarine, melted
1 teaspoon vanilla extract
⅓ cup carob powder
6 French bread slices (cut ¾ inch thick and one
   inch square)
1 teaspoon powdered cinnamon

In a large bowl, combine the low-fat milk, egg substitute, Prune Purée, sugar substitute, evaporated skim milk, margarine, vanilla extract and carob powder. Blend very well. Add the bread cubes and mix. Place the mixture in 8 8-ounce pudding cups. Cover and place in the refrigerator for 3 hours.

Preheat oven to 350° F. Uncover the pudding cups. Bake for 45 minutes. Sprinkle the tops with cinnamon. Serve immediately. Yield: 8 servings.

Nutritional Values (per serving)

Calories:	161	Fiber:	2.44 g
Carbohydrates:	22.5 g	Protein:	9.59 g
Cholesterol:	1.99 mg	Sodium:	279 mg
Fat:	3.38 g		

APPENDIX: COMPLETE NUTRITIONAL VALUES

⑨ After Dinner Mints

Calories	1.56
Protein	.084 g
Carbohydrates	.119 g
Fat—Total	.085 g
Saturated Fat	.053 g
Monounsaturated Fat	.024 g
Polyunsaturated Fat	.003 g
Omega 3 Fatty Acid	.001 g
Omega 6 Fatty Acid	.002 g
Cholesterol	.346 mg
Dietary Fiber	0 g
Total Vitamin A	.788 RE
A–Retinol	.686 RE
A–Carotenoid	.076 RE
Thiamin–B1	.001 mg
Riboflavin–B2	.004 mg
Niacin–B3	.002 mg
Niacin Equivalent	.002 mg
Vitamin B6	.001 mg
Vitamin B12	.009 mcg
Folate	.127 mcg
Pantothenic	.008 mg
Vitamin C	.024 mg
Vitamin D	.025 mcg
Vitamin E-Alpha E	.002 mg

Calcium	3.02 mg
Copper	0 mg
Iron	.001 mg
Magnesium	.341 mg
Manganese	0 mg
Phosphorus	2.38 mg
Potassium	3.86 mg
Selenium	.051 mcg
Sodium	1.25 mg
Zinc	.01 mg
Complex Carbohydrates	0 g
Sugars	.119 g
Mono-Saccharide	0 g
Di-Saccharide	.119 g
Alcohol	0 g
Caffeine	0 mg
Water	2.24 g

⊚ Almond Balls

Calories	72.2
Protein	2.08 g
Carbohydrates	9.62 g
Fat—Total	2.9 g
Saturated Fat	1.1 g
Monounsaturated Fat	1.06 g
Polyunsaturated Fat	.5 g
Omega 3 Fatty Acid	.015 g
Omega 6 Fatty Acid	.484 g
Cholesterol	7.63 mg
Dietary Fiber	.631 g
Total Vitamin A	14.4 RE
A–Retinol	13.1 RE
A–Carotenoid	.97 RE
Thiamin–B1	.067 mg
Riboflavin–B2	.065 mg
Niacin–B3	.606 mg
Niacin Equivalent	.603 mg
Vitamin B6	.04 mg
Vitamin B12	.028 mcg
Folate	6.69 mcg
Pantothenic	.132 mg
Vitamin C	.893 mg
Vitamin D	.054 mcg
Vitamin E-Alpha E	.591 mg

Calcium	37.5 mg
Copper	.045 mg
Iron	.526 mg
Magnesium	9.45 mg
Manganese	.128 mg
Phosphorus	27.4 mg
Potassium	71.3 mg
Selenium	2.85 mcg
Sodium	4.61 mg
Zinc	.163 mg
Complex Carbohydrates	6.35 g
Sugars	1.81 g
Mono-Saccharide	.075 g
Di-Saccharide	.267 g
Alcohol	0 g
Caffeine	0 mg
Water	13.5 g

☺ Almond Delight

Calories	28.9
Protein	1.09 g
Carbohydrates	.909 g
Fat—Total	2.54 g
Saturated Fat	.241 g
Monounsaturated Fat	1.65 g
Polyunsaturated Fat	.533 g
Omega 3 Fatty Acid	.018 g
Omega 6 Fatty Acid	.513 g
Cholesterol	0 mg
Dietary Fiber	.474 g
Total Vitamin A	.002 RE
A–Retinol	0 RE
A–Carotenoid	.002 RE
Thiamin–B1	.008 mg
Riboflavin–B2	.037 mg
Niacin–B3	.154 mg
Niacin Equivalent	.155 mg
Vitamin B6	.005 mg
Vitamin B12	.002 mcg
Folate	1.9 mcg
Pantothenic	.024 mg
Vitamin C	.072 mg
Vitamin D	0 mcg
Vitamin E-Alpha E	.271 mg

Calcium	12 mg
Copper	.052 mg
Iron	.177 mg
Magnesium	13.9 mg
Manganese	.07 mg
Phosphorus	25.8 mg
Potassium	37.7 mg
Selenium	.408 mcg
Sodium	2.15 mg
Zinc	.154 mg
Complex Carbohydrates	.156 g
Sugars	.281 g
Mono-Saccharide	.011 g
Di-Saccharide	0 g
Alcohol	0 g
Caffeine	0 mg
Water	1.18 g

⑨ Almond Pound Cake

Calories	56.8
Protein	1.95 g
Carbohydrates	8.82 g
Fat—Total	1.47 g
Saturated Fat	.281 g
Monounsaturated Fat	.519 g
Polyunsaturated Fat	.541 g
Omega 3 Fatty Acid	.01 g
Omega 6 Fatty Acid	.533 g
Cholesterol	10.7 mg
Dietary Fiber	.358 g
Total Vitamin A	35.5 RE
A–Retinol	33.1 RE
A–Carotenoid	2.32 RE
Thiamin–B1	.089 mg
Riboflavin–B2	.088 mg
Niacin–B3	.655 mg
Niacin Equivalent	.655 mg
Vitamin B6	.01 mg
Vitamin B12	.049 mcg
Folate	4.35 mcg
Pantothenic	.098 mg
Vitamin C	.043 mg
Vitamin D	.375 mcg
Vitamin E-Alpha E	.239 mg

Calcium	27.2 mg
Copper	.017 mg
Iron	.582 mg
Magnesium	3.66 mg
Manganese	.077 mg
Phosphorus	50.7 mg
Potassium	70.4 mg
Selenium	5.15 mcg
Sodium	21.3 mg
Zinc	.124 mg
Complex Carbohydrates	8 g
Sugars	.463 g
Mono-Saccharide	.164 g
Di-Saccharide	.242 g
Alcohol	0 g
Caffeine	0 mg
Water	11.5 g

☺ Apple Pie

Calories	71.2
Protein	.377 g
Carbohydrates	18.2 g
Fat—Total	.415 g
Saturated Fat	.067 g
Monounsaturated Fat	.018 g
Polyunsaturated Fat	.124 g
Omega 3 Fatty Acid	.021 g
Omega 6 Fatty Acid	.103 g
Cholesterol	0 mg
Dietary Fiber	2.23 g
Total Vitamin A	5.88 RE
A–Retinol	0 RE
A–Carotenoid	5.88 RE
Thiamin–B1	.031 mg
Riboflavin–B2	.023 mg
Niacin–B3	.179 mg
Niacin Equivalent	.177 mg
Vitamin B6	.054 mg
Vitamin B12	0 mcg
Folate	3.69 mcg
Pantothenic	.076 mg
Vitamin C	7 mg
Vitamin D	0 mcg
Vitamin E-Alpha E	.658 mg

Calcium	8.07 mg
Copper	.048 mg
Iron	.271 mg
Magnesium	5.95 mg
Manganese	.06 mg
Phosphorus	9.51 mg
Potassium	131 mg
Selenium	.864 mcg
Sodium	.047 mg
Zinc	.056 mg
Complex Carbohydrates	1.12 g
Sugars	13.4 g
Mono-Saccharide	9.25 g
Di-Saccharide	2.88 g
Alcohol	0 g
Caffeine	0 mg
Water	94.2 g

⊚ Apple-Raisin Surprise

Calories	38.3
Protein	.874 g
Carbohydrates	3.38 g
Fat—Total	2.65 g
Saturated Fat	.717 g
Monounsaturated Fat	1.38 g
Polyunsaturated Fat	.425 g
Omega 3 Fatty Acid	.012 g
Omega 6 Fatty Acid	.411 g
Cholesterol	0 mg
Dietary Fiber	.487 g
Total Vitamin A	.051 RE
A–Retinol	0 RE
A–Carotenoid	.051 RE
Thiamin–B1	.012 mg
Riboflavin–B2	.024 mg
Niacin–B3	.136 mg
Niacin Equivalent	.137 mg
Vitamin B6	.015 mg
Vitamin B12	0 mcg
Folate	3.34 mcg
Pantothenic	.053 mg
Vitamin C	.126 mg
Vitamin D	0 mcg
Vitamin E-Alpha E	.549 mg

Calcium	7.98 mg
Copper	.082 mg
Iron	.292 mg
Magnesium	13.6 mg
Manganese	.097 mg
Phosphorus	25.4 mg
Potassium	53.4 mg
Selenium	.965 mcg
Sodium	1.55 mg
Zinc	.213 mg
Complex Carbohydrates	.631 g
Sugars	2.22 g
Mono-Saccharide	.443 g
Di-Saccharide	.582 g
Alcohol	0 g
Caffeine	0 mg
Water	2.36 g

⑨ Applesauce-Pineapple Cake

Calories	105
Protein	1.27 g
Carbohydrates	9.58 g
Fat—Total	7.29 g
Saturated Fat	.925 g
Monounsaturated Fat	2.26 g
Polyunsaturated Fat	3.75 g
Omega 3 Fatty Acid	.427 g
Omega 6 Fatty Acid	3.3 g
Cholesterol	.177 mg
Dietary Fiber	.544 g
Total Vitamin A	71.6 RE
A–Retinol	64.5 RE
A–Carotenoid	6.88 RE
Thiamin–B1	.045 mg
Riboflavin–B2	.032 mg
Niacin–B3	.254 mg
Niacin Equivalent	.254 mg
Vitamin B6	.045 mg
Vitamin B12	0.15 mcg
Folate	5.13 mcg
Pantothenic	.087 mg
Vitamin C	1.06 mg
Vitamin D	.755 mcg
Vitamin E-Alpha E	.614 mg

Calcium	19.1 mg
Copper	.092 mg
Iron	.3 mg
Magnesium	11.5 mg
Manganese	.267 mg
Phosphorus	47.2 mg
Potassium	49.4 mg
Selenium	.355 mcg
Sodium	84 mg
Zinc	.185 mg
Complex Carbohydrates	.949 g
Sugars	8.05 g
Mono-Saccharide	.242 g
Di-Saccharide	.268 g
Alcohol	0 g
Caffeine	0 mg
Water	16.7 g

☺ Apricot Balls

Calories	10.8
Protein	.175 g
Carbohydrates	1.16 g
Fat—Total	.7 g
Saturated Fat	.597 g
Monounsaturated Fat	.041 g
Polyunsaturated Fat	.013 g
Omega 3 Fatty Acid	0 g
Omega 6 Fatty Acid	.013 g
Cholesterol	0 mg
Dietary Fiber	.324 g
Total Vitamin A	19.8 RE
A–Retinol	0 RE
A–Carotenoid	19.8 RE
Thiamin–B1	.004 mg
Riboflavin–B2	.003 mg
Niacin–B3	.057 mg
Niacin Equivalent	.057 mg
Vitamin B6	.005 mg
Vitamin B12	0 mcg
Folate	1.23 mcg
Pantothenic	.024 mg
Vitamin C	.908 mg
Vitamin D	.0 mcg
Vitamin E-Alpha E	.082 mg

Calcium	1.36 mg
Copper	.016 mg
Iron	.09 mg
Magnesium	1.26 mg
Manganese	.036 mg
Phosphorus	3.73 mg
Potassium	29.9 mg
Selenium	.494 mcg
Sodium	.477 mg
Zinc	.042 mg
Complex Carbohydrates	0 g
Sugars	.8 g
Mono-Saccharide	.252 g
Di-Saccharide	.478 g
Alcohol	0 g
Caffeine	0 mg
Water	7.62 g

☺ Avocado Pie

Calories	238
Protein	4.91 g
Carbohydrates	27 g
Fat—Total	13.4 g
Saturated Fat	5.38 g
Monounsaturated Fat	5.92 g
Polyunsaturated Fat	1.17 g
Omega 3 Fatty Acid	.124 g
Omega 6 Fatty Acid	1.04 g
Cholesterol	13 mg
Dietary Fiber	2.08 g
Total Vitamin A	69.9 RE
A–Retinol	27.9 RE
A–Carotenoid	42 RE
Thiamin–B1	.09 mg
Riboflavin–B2	.222 mg
Niacin–B3	1.05 mg
Niacin Equivalent	1.05 mg
Vitamin B6	.162 mg
Vitamin B12	.17 mcg
Folate	36.1 mcg
Pantothenic	.781 mg
Vitamin C	6.73 mg
Vitamin D	.045 mcg
Vitamin E-Alpha E	1.24 mg

Calcium	115 mg
Copper	.161 mg
Iron	.613 mg
Magnesium	30 mg
Manganese	.123 mg
Phosphorus	119 mg
Potassium	450 mg
Selenium	.656 mcg
Sodium	57.8 mg
Zinc	.577 mg
Complex Carbohydrates	1.21 g
Sugars	23.7 g
Mono-Saccharide	.433 g
Di-Saccharide	20.8 g
Alcohol	0 g
Caffeine	0 mg
Water	56.1 g

☻ Banana Cookies

Calories	29.2
Protein	.698 g
Carbohydrates	4.82 g
Fat—Total	.851 g
Saturated Fat	.131 g
Monounsaturated Fat	.259 g
Polyunsaturated Fat	.283 g
Omega 3 Fatty Acid	.005 g
Omega 6 Fatty Acid	.279 g
Cholesterol	2.96 mg
Dietary Fiber	.275 g
Total Vitamin A	26.5 RE
A–Retinol	15.7 RE
A–Carotenoid	1.37 RE
Thiamin–B1	.055 mg
Riboflavin–B2	.051 mg
Niacin–B3	.552 mg
Niacin Equivalent	.237 mg
Vitamin B6	.04 mg
Vitamin B12	.103 mcg
Folate	7.87 mcg
Pantothenic	.029 mg
Vitamin C	.096 mg
Vitamin D	.24 mcg
Vitamin E-Alpha E	.121 mg

Calcium	1.27 mg
Copper	.012 mg
Iron	.308 mg
Magnesium	2.77 mg
Manganese	.028 mg
Phosphorus	10.9 mg
Potassium	15.5 mg
Selenium	1.94 mcg
Sodium	10.3 mg
Zinc	.273 mg
Complex Carbohydrates	3.7 g
Sugars	.842 g
Mono-Saccharide	.123 g
Di-Saccharide	.124 g
Alcohol	0 g
Caffeine	0 mg
Water	2.74 g

☺ Blueberry Cake

Calories	68.6
Protein	1.47 g
Carbohydrates	7.96 g
Fat—Total	3.52 g
Saturated Fat	1.78 g
Monounsaturated Fat	.775 g
Polyunsaturated Fat	.701 g
Omega 3 Fatty Acid	.013 g
Omega 6 Fatty Acid	.679 g
Cholesterol	20 mg
Dietary Fiber	.684 g
Total Vitamin A	46.2 RE
A–Retinol	41.2 RE
A–Carotenoid	4.9 RE
Thiamin–B1	.081 mg
Riboflavin–B2	.064 mg
Niacin–B3	.575 mg
Niacin Equivalent	.575 mg
Vitamin B6	.021 mg
Vitamin B12	.049 mcg
Folate	6.51 mcg
Pantothenic	.134 mg
Vitamin C	4.51 mg
Vitamin D	.438 mcg
Vitamin E-Alpha E	.354 mg

Calcium	5.74 mg
Copper	.037 mg
Iron	.722 mg
Magnesium	5 mg
Manganese	.13 mg
Phosphorus	22 mg
Potassium	47.2 mg
Selenium	2.22 mcg
Sodium	19.8 mg
Zinc	.157 mg
Complex Carbohydrates	5.59 g
Sugars	1.7 g
Mono-Saccharide	.83 g
Di-Saccharide	.328 g
Alcohol	0 g
Caffeine	0 mg
Water	17.3 g

⊚ Bon Bons

Calories	31.4
Protein	.968 g
Carbohydrates	3.86 g
Fat—Total	1.39 g
Saturated Fat	1.18 g
Monounsaturated Fat	.041 g
Polyunsaturated Fat	.005 g
Omega 3 Fatty Acid	.002 g
Omega 6 Fatty Acid	.003 g
Cholesterol	.916 mg
Dietary Fiber	.003 g
Total Vitamin A	1.91 RE
A–Retinol	1.4 RE
A–Carotenoid	.155 RE
Thiamin–B1	.002 mg
Riboflavin–B2	.009 mg
Niacin–B3	.003 mg
Niacin Equivalent	.003 mg
Vitamin B6	.002 mg
Vitamin B12	.022 mcg
Folate	.198 mcg
Pantothenic	.017 mg
Vitamin C	.026 mg
Vitamin D	.002 mcg
Vitamin E-Alpha E	.004 mg

Calcium	40.5 mg
Copper	0 mg
Iron	.055 mg
Magnesium	.495 mg
Manganese	0 mg
Phosphorus	3.6 mg
Potassium	6.95 mg
Selenium	.126 mcg
Sodium	2.81 mg
Zinc	.015 mg
Complex Carbohydrates	.003 g
Sugars	2.7 g
Mono-Saccharide	0 g
Di-Saccharide	0 g
Alcohol	0 g
Caffeine	0 mg
Water	2.25 g

⑨ Bread Pudding

Calories	161
Protein	9.59 g
Carbohydrates	22.5 g
Fat—Total	3.38 g
Saturated Fat	.696 g
Monounsaturated Fat	1.16 g
Polyunsaturated Fat	1.28 g
Omega 3 Fatty Acid	.075 g
Omega 6 Fatty Acid	1.2 g
Cholesterol	1.99 mg
Dietary Fiber	2.44 g
Total Vitamin A	159 RE
A–Retinol	88.1 RE
A–Carotenoid	70.7 RE
Thiamin–B1	.203 mg
Riboflavin–B2	.336 mg
Niacin–B3	1.44 mg
Niacin Equivalent	1.45 mg
Vitamin B6	.061 mg
Vitamin B12	.365 mcg
Folate	18.7 mcg
Pantothenic	1.27 mg
Vitamin C	.811 mg
Vitamin D	1.61 mcg
Vitamin E-Alpha E	.535 mg

Calcium	173 mg
Copper	.091 mg
Iron	1.52 mg
Magnesium	23.5 mg
Manganese	.16 mg
Phosphorus	162 mg
Potassium	324 mg
Selenium	10.2 mcg
Sodium	279 mg
Zinc	1.07 mg
Complex Carbohydrates	12.6 g
Sugars	5.32 g
Mono-Saccharide	0 g
Di-Saccharide	4.79 g
Alcohol	0 g
Caffeine	0 mg
Water	105 g

⊚ Brownies

Calories	38.2
Protein	.852 g
Carbohydrates	4.03 g
Fat—Total	2.09 g
Saturated Fat	.655 g
Monounsaturated Fat	.325 g
Polyunsaturated Fat	1.01 g
Omega 3 Fatty Acid	.006 g
Omega 6 Fatty Acid	1 g
Cholesterol	.292 mg
Dietary Fiber	.626 g
Total Vitamin A	.439 RE
A–Retinol	.238 RE
A–Carotenoid	.048 RE
Thiamin–B1	.015 mg
Riboflavin–B2	.026 mg
Niacin–B3	.133 mg
Niacin Equivalent	.133 mg
Vitamin B6	.007 mg
Vitamin B12	.013 mcg
Folate	1.1 mcg
Pantothenic	.02 mg
Vitamin C	.016 mg
Vitamin D	.001 mcg
Vitamin E-Alpha E	.919 mg

Calcium	23.4 mg
Copper	.011 mg
Iron	.146 mg
Magnesium	1.63 mg
Manganese	.019 mg
Phosphorus	5.66 mg
Potassium	19.9 mg
Selenium	1.03 mcg
Sodium	4.32 mg
Zinc	.041 mg
Complex Carbohydrates	1.24 g
Sugars	.979 g
Mono-Saccharide	.061 g
Di-Saccharide	.085 g
Alcohol	0 g
Caffeine	0 mg
Water	3.09 g

⊚ Buckeyes

Calories	61.2
Protein	2.1 g
Carbohydrates	2.63 g
Fat—Total	5.06 g
Saturated Fat	1.39 g
Monounsaturated Fat	1.98 g
Polyunsaturated Fat	1.25 g
Omega 3 Fatty Acid	.009 g
Omega 6 Fatty Acid	1.24 g
Cholesterol	.242 mg
Dietary Fiber	.399 g
Total Vitamin A	15.2 RE
A–Retinol	13.8 RE
A–Carotenoid	1.24 RE
Thiamin–B1	.01 mg
Riboflavin–B2	.006 mg
Niacin–B3	.858 mg
Niacin Equivalent	.858 mg
Vitamin B6	.027 mg
Vitamin B12	.001 mcg
Folate	4.74 mcg
Pantothenic	.056 mg
Vitamin C	.001 mg
Vitamin D	0 mcg
Vitamin E-Alpha E	.194 mg

Calcium	21.5 mg
Copper	.039 mg
Iron	.142 mg
Magnesium	10.9 mg
Manganese	.097 mg
Phosphorus	21.4 mg
Potassium	42.3 mg
Selenium	0 mcg
Sodium	1.06 mg
Zinc	.181 mg
Complex Carbohydrates	.376 g
Sugars	1.52 g
Mono-Saccharide	.073 g
Di-Saccharide	.399 g
Alcohol	0 g
Caffeine	0 mg
Water	.353 g

⊚ Butter Crunch

Calories	28.4
Protein	.339 g
Carbohydrates	.348 g
Fat—Total	2.96 g
Saturated Fat	.521 g
Monounsaturated Fat	1.38 g
Polyunsaturated Fat	.925 g
Omega 3 Fatty Acid	.009 g
Omega 6 Fatty Acid	.917 g
Cholesterol	0 mg
Dietary Fiber	.095 g
Total Vitamin A	28.2 RE
A–Retinol	25.8 RE
A–Carotenoid	2.32 RE
Thiamin–B1	.006 mg
Riboflavin–B2	.002 mg
Niacin–B3	.185 mg
Niacin Equivalent	.185 mg
Vitamin B6	.004 mg
Vitamin B12	.002 mcg
Folate	2.01 mcg
Pantothenic	.021 mg
Vitamin C	.003 mg
Vitamin D	0 mcg
Vitamin E-Alpha E	.465 mg

Calcium	1.23 mg
Copper	.009 mg
Iron	.031 mg
Magnesium	2.44 mg
Manganese	.029 mg
Phosphorus	5.32 mg
Potassium	9.71 mg
Selenium	.101 mcg
Sodium	.322 mg
Zinc	.045 mg
Complex Carbohydrates	.137 g
Sugars	.077 g
Mono-Saccharide	.003 g
Di-Saccharide	.055 g
Alcohol	0 g
Caffeine	0 mg
Water	.595 g

❾ Candied Nuts

Calories	40.9
Protein	.636 g
Carbohydrates	4.17 g
Fat—Total	2.75 g
Saturated Fat	.248 g
Monounsaturated Fat	.631 g
Polyunsaturated Fat	1.74 g
Omega 3 Fatty Acid	.303 g
Omega 6 Fatty Acid	1.41 g
Cholesterol	0 mg
Dietary Fiber	.201 g
Total Vitamin A	.551 RE
A–Retinol	0 RE
A–Carotenoid	.551 RE
Thiamin–B1	.018 mg
Riboflavin–B2	.007 mg
Niacin–B3	.048 mg
Niacin Equivalent	.048 mg
Vitamin B6	.025 mg
Vitamin B12	0 mcg
Folate	2.93 mcg
Pantothenic	.03 mg
Vitamin C	.143 mg
Vitamin D	0 mcg
Vitamin E-Alpha E	.116 mg

Calcium	4.25 mg
Copper	.062 mg
Iron	.11 mg
Magnesium	7.51 mg
Manganese	.136 mg
Phosphorus	17.3 mg
Potassium	22.5 mg
Selenium	.222 mcg
Sodium	15.6 mg
Zinc	.123 mg
Complex Carbohydrates	.52 g
Sugars	.097 g
Mono-Saccharide	0 g
Di-Saccharide	.093 g
Alcohol	0 g
Caffeine	0 mg
Water	4.31 g

⊘ Candied Prunes

Calories	13.7
Protein	.148 g
Carbohydrates	3.6 g
Fat—Total	.029 g
Saturated Fat	.002 g
Monounsaturated Fat	.019 g
Polyunsaturated Fat	.006 g
Omega 3 Fatty Acid	0 g
Omega 6 Fatty Acid	.006 g
Cholesterol	0 mg
Dietary Fiber	.524 g
Total Vitamin A	11.3 RE
A–Retinol	0 RE
A–Carotenoid	11.3 RE
Thiamin–B1	.005 mg
Riboflavin–B2	.009 mg
Niacin–B3	.111 mg
Niacin Equivalent	.111 mg
Vitamin B6	.015 mg
Vitamin B12	0 mcg
Folate	.21 mcg
Pantothenic	.026 mg
Vitamin C	.187 mg
Vitamin D	0 mcg
Vitamin E-Alpha E	.076 mg

Calcium	2.93 mg
Copper	.025 mg
Iron	.146 mg
Magnesium	2.72 mg
Manganese	.013 mg
Phosphorus	4.55 mg
Potassium	43 mg
Selenium	.152 mcg
Sodium	.234 mg
Zinc	.03 mg
Complex Carbohydrates	0 g
Sugars	2.48 g
Mono-Saccharide	2.11 g
Di-Saccharide	.045 g
Alcohol	0 g
Caffeine	0 mg
Water	2.54 g

☺ Carob Chip Cookies

Calories	59
Protein	1.76 g
Carbohydrates	7.33 g
Fat—Total	2.52 g
Saturated Fat	1.67 g
Monounsaturated Fat	.285 g
Polyunsaturated Fat	.292 g
Omega 3 Fatty Acid	.005 g
Omega 6 Fatty Acid	.288 g
Cholesterol	6.55 mg
Dietary Fiber	.128 g
Total Vitamin A	18.8 RE
A–Retinol	17 RE
A–Carotenoid	1.29 RE
Thiamin–B1	.032 mg
Riboflavin–B2	.027 mg
Niacin–B3	.232 mg
Niacin Equivalent	.232 mg
Vitamin B6	.004 mg
Vitamin B12	.015 mcg
Folate	1.68 mcg
Pantothenic	.035 mg
Vitamin C	.002 mg
Vitamin D	.186 mcg
Vitamin E-Alpha E	.125 mg

Calcium	51.4 mg
Copper	.006 mg
Iron	.273 mg
Magnesium	1.02 mg
Manganese	.027 mg
Phosphorus	6.91 mg
Potassium	6.27 mg
Selenium	1.75 mcg
Sodium	7.38 mg
Zinc	.043 mg
Complex Carbohydrates	2.78 g
Sugars	2.8 g
Mono-Saccharide	.052 g
Di-Saccharide	.016 g
Alcohol	0 g
Caffeine	0 mg
Water	2.43 g

◉ Carob and Coconut Macaroons

Calories	56.1
Protein	1.28 g
Carbohydrates	3.56 g
Fat—Total	4.33 g
Saturated Fat	3.69 g
Monounsaturated Fat	.23 g
Polyunsaturated Fat	.068 g
Omega 3 Fatty Acid	.002 g
Omega 6 Fatty Acid	.067 g
Cholesterol	11 mg
Dietary Fiber	.838 g
Total Vitamin A	5.05 RE
A–Retinol	4.78 RE
A–Carotenoid	0 RE
Thiamin–B1	.004 mg
Riboflavin–B2	.018 mg
Niacin–B3	.031 mg
Niacin Equivalent	.031 mg
Vitamin B6	.018 mg
Vitamin B12	.025 mcg
Folate	1.61 mcg
Pantothenic	.07 mg
Vitamin C	.074 mg
Vitamin D	.032 mcg
Vitamin E-Alpha E	.091 mg

Calcium	29.4 mg
Copper	.039 mg
Iron	.238 mg
Magnesium	4.64 mg
Manganese	.135 mg
Phosphorus	14.5 mg
Potassium	33 mg
Selenium	1.55 mcg
Sodium	4.97 mg
Zinc	.127 mg
Complex Carbohydrates	.013 g
Sugars	1.88 g
Mono-Saccharide	.031 g
Di-Saccharide	0 g
Alcohol	0 g
Caffeine	0 mg
Water	2.03 g

☺ Carrott Cake

Calories	35.9
Protein	.829 g
Carbohydrates	8.02 g
Fat—Total	.095 g
Saturated Fat	.017 g
Monounsaturated Fat	.008 g
Polyunsaturated Fat	.036 g
Omega 3 Fatty Acid	.004 g
Omega 6 Fatty Acid	.032 g
Cholesterol	.022 mg
Dietary Fiber	.496 g
Total Vitamin A	125 RE
A–Retinol	.745 RE
A–Carotenoid	124 RE
Thiamin–B1	.063 mg
Riboflavin–B2	.041 mg
Niacin–B3	.46 mg
Niacin Equivalent	.459 mg
Vitamin B6	.023 mg
Vitamin B12	.005 mcg
Folate	2.83 mcg
Pantothenic	.052 mg
Vitamin C	1.26 mg
Vitamin D	.012 mcg
Vitamin E-Alpha E	.071 mg

Calcium	7.04 mg
Copper	.028 mg
Iron	.417 mg
Magnesium	4.42 mg
Manganese	.18 mg
Phosphorus	12.6 mg
Potassium	46.3 mg
Selenium	2.44 mcg
Sodium	52.9 mg
Zinc	.077 mg
Complex Carbohydrates	4.51 g
Sugars	3.02 g
Mono-Saccharide	1.22 g
Di-Saccharide	.243 g
Alcohol	0 g
Caffeine	0 mg
Water	14.7 g

☺ Cherries à la Fudge

Calories	33.5
Protein	1.13 g
Carbohydrates	4.53 g
Fat—Total	1.25 g
Saturated Fat	1.1 g
Monounsaturated Fat	.002 g
Polyunsaturated Fat	.002 g
Omega 3 Fatty Acid	.001 g
Omega 6 Fatty Acid	.001 g
Cholesterol	.454 mg
Dietary Fiber	0 g
Total Vitamin A	.365 RE
A–Retinol	0 RE
A–Carotenoid	0 RE
Thiamin–B1	0 mg
Riboflavin–B2	.001 mg
Niacin–B3	0 mg
Niacin Equivalent	0 mg
Vitamin B6	0 mg
Vitamin B12	0 mcg
Folate	.07 mcg
Pantothenic	0 mg
Vitamin C	0 mg
Vitamin D	0 mcg
Vitamin E-Alpha E	.006 mg

Calcium	36.5 mg
Copper	.005 mg
Iron	.064 mg
Magnesium	.005 mg
Manganese	0 mg
Phosphorus	7 mg
Potassium	5.43 mg
Selenium	0 mcg
Sodium	10.9 mg
Zinc	0 mg
Complex Carbohydrates	0 g
Sugars	1.95 g
Mono-Saccharide	0 g
Di-Saccharide	0 g
Alcohol	0 g
Caffeine	0 mg
Water	3.01 g

⊘ Cherry Cheesecake

Calories	66.3
Protein	4.37 g
Carbohydrates	12 g
Fat—Total	.129 g
Saturated Fat	.058 g
Monounsaturated Fat	.036 g
Polyunsaturated Fat	.022 g
Omega 3 Fatty Acid	.009 g
Omega 6 Fatty Acid	.013 g
Cholesterol	2.82 mg
Dietary Fiber	.416 g
Total Vitamin A	101 RE
A–Retinol	43.1 RE
A–Carotenoid	34.3 RE
Thiamin–B1	.026 mg
Riboflavin–B2	.15 mg
Niacin–B3	.151 mg
Niacin Equivalent	.145 mg
Vitamin B6	.043 mg
Vitamin B12	.088 mcg
Folate	7.58 mcg
Pantothenic	.326 mg
Vitamin C	4.21 mg
Vitamin D	.737 mcg
Vitamin E-Alpha E	.035 mg

Calcium	112 mg
Copper	.041 mg
Iron	.75 mg
Magnesium	13.1 mg
Manganese	.039 mg
Phosphorus	77.1 mg
Potassium	175 mg
Selenium	1.23 mcg
Sodium	96.8 mg
Zinc	.369 mg
Complex Carbohydrates	2.89 g
Sugars	8.41 g
Mono-Saccharide	.128 g
Di-Saccharide	4.22 g
Alcohol	0 g
Caffeine	0 mg
Water	75.9 g

⑨ Cherry Fudge

Calories	34.6
Protein	.231 g
Carbohydrates	.651 g
Fat—Total	3.56 g
Saturated Fat	.747 g
Monounsaturated Fat	1.45 g
Polyunsaturated Fat	1.2 g
Omega 3 Fatty Acid	.075 g
Omega 6 Fatty Acid	1.12 g
Cholesterol	.992 mg
Dietary Fiber	.043 g
Total Vitamin A	36.5 RE
A–Retinol	33.1 RE
A–Carotenoid	3.31 RE
Thiamin–B1	.005 mg
Riboflavin–B2	.006 mg
Niacin–B3	.014 mg
Niacin Equivalent	.014 mg
Vitamin B6	.007 mg
Vitamin B12	.011 mcg
Folate	.854 mcg
Pantothenic	.016 mg
Vitamin C	.399 mg
Vitamin D	.011 mcg
Vitamin E-Alpha E	.465 mg

Calcium	4.52 mg
Copper	.013 mg
Iron	.028 mg
Magnesium	1.9 mg
Manganese	.026 mg
Phosphorus	6.04 mg
Potassium	13.5 mg
Selenium	.094 mcg
Sodium	1.28 mg
Zinc	.038 mg
Complex Carbohydrates	.122 g
Sugars	.208 g
Mono-Saccharide	.031 g
Di-Saccharide	.156 g
Alcohol	0 g
Caffeine	0 mg
Water	4.02 g

◉ Cherry Coconut Macaroons

Calories	34.1
Protein	.546 g
Carbohydrates	1.26 g
Fat—Total	3.23 g
Saturated Fat	2.87 g
Monounsaturated Fat	.138 g
Polyunsaturated Fat	.035 g
Omega 3 Fatty Acid	0 g
Omega 6 Fatty Acid	.035 g
Cholesterol	0 mg
Dietary Fiber	.862 g
Total Vitamin A	0 RE
A–Retinol	0 RE
A–Carotenoid	0 RE
Thiamin–B1	.003 mg
Riboflavin–B2	.014 mg
Niacin–B3	.032 mg
Niacin Equivalent	.032 mg
Vitamin B6	.015 mg
Vitamin B12	.004 mcg
Folate	.509 mcg
Pantothenic	.042 mg
Vitamin C	.076 mg
Vitamin D	0 mcg
Vitamin E-Alpha E	.07 mg

Calcium	1.42 mg
Copper	.04 mg
Iron	.169 mg
Magnesium	4.72 mg
Manganese	.138 mg
Phosphorus	10.6 mg
Potassium	33.9 mg
Selenium	1.14 mcg
Sodium	5 mg
Zinc	.102 mg
Complex Carbohydrates	.014 g
Sugars	.416 g
Mono-Saccharide	.02 g
Di-Saccharide	0 g
Alcohol	0 g
Caffeine	0 mg
Water	1.83 g

☺ Cherry Scones

Calories	110
Protein	2.75 g
Carbohydrates	21.1 g
Fat—Total	2.73 g
Saturated Fat	.4 g
Monounsaturated Fat	.665 g
Polyunsaturated Fat	1.5 g
Omega 3 Fatty Acid	.015 g
Omega 6 Fatty Acid	1.49 g
Cholesterol	.56 mg
Dietary Fiber	1.05 g
Total Vitamin A	68.6 RE
A–Retinol	21.5 RE
A–Carotenoid	2.45 RE
Thiamin–B1	.129 mg
Riboflavin–B2	.119 mg
Niacin–B3	.949 mg
Niacin Equivalent	.893 mg
Vitamin B6	.017 mg
Vitamin B12	.046 mcg
Folate	5.07 mcg
Pantothenic	.165 mg
Vitamin C	.273 mg
Vitamin D	.27 mcg
Vitamin E-Alpha E	1.19 mg

Calcium	46.8 mg
Copper	.072 mg
Iron	.881 mg
Magnesium	12.5 mg
Manganese	.145 mg
Phosphorus	72.1 mg
Potassium	105 mg
Selenium	5.68 mcg
Sodium	21.8 mg
Zinc	.245 mg
Complex Carbohydrates	11.3 g
Sugars	1.1 g
Mono-Saccharide	.248 g
Di-Saccharide	.743 g
Alcohol	0 g
Caffeine	0 mg
Water	15.6 g

◎ Chocolate Bars

Calories	54.2
Protein	1.35 g
Carbohydrates	6.12 g
Fat—Total	2.72 g
Saturated Fat	1.45 g
Monounsaturated Fat	.488 g
Polyunsaturated Fat	.537 g
Omega 3 Fatty Acid	.008 g
Omega 6 Fatty Acid	.532 g
Cholesterol	3.46 mg
Dietary Fiber	.114 g
Total Vitamin A	33.1 RE
A–Retinol	30 RE
A–Carotenoid	2.58 RE
Thiamin–B1	.028 mg
Riboflavin–B2	.019 mg
Niacin–B3	.205 mg
Niacin Equivalent	.205 mg
Vitamin B6	.003 mg
Vitamin B12	.009 mcg
Folate	1.26 mcg
Pantothenic	.026 mg
Vitamin C	.003 mg
Vitamin D	.344 mcg
Vitamin E-Alpha E	.215 mg

Calcium	41.3 mg
Copper	.005 mg
Iron	.227 mg
Magnesium	.834 mg
Manganese	.024 mg
Phosphorus	5.31 mg
Potassium	4.74 mg
Selenium	1.28 mcg
Sodium	11.3 mg
Zinc	.031 mg
Complex Carbohydrates	2.48 g
Sugars	2.24 g
Mono-Saccharide	.036 g
Di-Saccharide	.014 g
Alcohol	0 g
Caffeine	0 mg
Water	2.36 g

◎ Chocolate Cake

Calories	54.3
Protein	1.47 g
Carbohydrates	7.95 g
Fat—Total	1.8 g
Saturated Fat	.222 g
Monounsaturated Fat	.367 g
Polyunsaturated Fat	1.16 g
Omega 3 Fatty Acid	.008 g
Omega 6 Fatty Acid	1.15 g
Cholesterol	.287 mg
Dietary Fiber	.736 g
Total Vitamin A	9.32 RE
A–Retinol	9.31 RE
A–Carotenoid	.012 RE
Thiamin–B1	.066 mg
Riboflavin–B2	.069 mg
Niacin–B3	.498 mg
Niacin Equivalent	.498 mg
Vitamin B6	.012 mg
Vitamin B12	.019 mcg
Folate	3.07 mcg
Pantothenic	.094 mg
Vitamin C	.102 mg
Vitamin D	.159 mcg
Vitamin E-Alpha E	1.05 mg

Calcium	28.5 mg
Copper	.019 mg
Iron	.422 mg
Magnesium	4.52 mg
Manganese	.06 mg
Phosphorus	24.9 mg
Potassium	44.8 mg
Selenium	2.93 mcg
Sodium	9.74 mg
Zinc	.138 mg
Complex Carbohydrates	5.57 g
Sugars	1.04 g
Mono-Saccharide	.071 g
Di-Saccharide	.941 g
Alcohol	0 g
Caffeine	0 mg
Water	7.3 g

☻ Chocolate Peanut Butter Fudge

Calories	33.5
Protein	1.12 g
Carbohydrates	3.37 g
Fat—Total	1.82 g
Saturated Fat	1.11 g
Monounsaturated Fat	.336 g
Polyunsaturated Fat	.206 g
Omega 3 Fatty Acid	.001 g
Omega 6 Fatty Acid	.204 g
Cholesterol	.403 mg
Dietary Fiber	.114 g
Total Vitamin A	.324 RE
A–Retinol	0 RE
A–Carotenoid	0 RE
Thiamin–B1	.003 mg
Riboflavin–B2	.002 mg
Niacin–B3	.214 mg
Niacin Equivalent	.214 mg
Vitamin B6	.01 mg
Vitamin B12	0 mcg
Folate	1.44 mcg
Pantothenic	.021 mg
Vitamin C	.111 mg
Vitamin D	0 mcg
Vitamin E-Alpha E	.107 mg

Calcium	32.6 mg
Copper	.01 mg
Iron	.077 mg
Magnesium	2.56 mg
Manganese	.029 mg
Phosphorus	5.09 mg
Potassium	15.5 mg
Selenium	.119 mcg
Sodium	.317 mg
Zinc	.044 mg
Complex Carbohydrates	.356 g
Sugars	1.86 g
Mono-Saccharide	.017 g
Di-Saccharide	.094 g
Alcohol	0 g
Caffeine	0 mg
Water	1.18 g

⑨ Chocolate Soufflé

Calories	40.2
Protein	.333 g
Carbohydrates	10.3 g
Fat—Total	.059 g
Saturated Fat	.005 g
Monounsaturated Fat	.035 g
Polyunsaturated Fat	.014 g
Omega 3 Fatty Acid	0 g
Omega 6 Fatty Acid	.014 g
Cholesterol	0 mg
Dietary Fiber	1.54 g
Total Vitamin A	18.8 RE
A–Retinol	0 RE
A–Carotenoid	18.8 RE
Thiamin–B1	.008 mg
Riboflavin–B2	.015 mg
Niacin–B3	.221 mg
Niacin Equivalent	.186 mg
Vitamin B6	.031 mg
Vitamin B12	0 mcg
Folate	.35 mcg
Pantothenic	.044 mg
Vitamin C	.312 mg
Vitamin D	0 mcg
Vitamin E-Alpha E	.126 mg

Calcium	6.33 mg
Copper	.043 mg
Iron	.453 mg
Magnesium	4.49 mg
Manganese	.024 mg
Phosphorus	7.8 mg
Potassium	75.3 mg
Selenium	.247 mcg
Sodium	5.26 mg
Zinc	.054 mg
Complex Carbohydrates	0 g
Sugars	4.06 g
Mono-Saccharide	3.51 g
Di-Saccharide	.076 g
Alcohol	0 g
Caffeine	0 mg
Water	3.2 g

❂ Christmas Trees

Calories	58.1
Protein	1.38 g
Carbohydrates	5.15 g
Fat—Total	3.68 g
Saturated Fat	2.79 g
Monounsaturated Fat	.371 g
Polyunsaturated Fat	.195 g
Omega 3 Fatty Acid	.004 g
Omega 6 Fatty Acid	.191 g
Cholesterol	1.51 mg
Dietary Fiber	.282 g
Total Vitamin A	9.8 RE
A–Retinol	8.5 RE
A–Carotenoid	.737 RE
Thiamin–B1	.002 mg
Riboflavin–B2	.002 mg
Niacin–B3	.017 mg
Niacin Equivalent	.017 mg
Vitamin B6	.002 mg
Vitamin B12	.002 mcg
Folate	.824 mcg
Pantothenic	.011 mg
Vitamin C	.105 mg
Vitamin D	.001 mcg
Vitamin E-Alpha E	.119 mg

Calcium	54.9 mg
Copper	.013 mg
Iron	.15 mg
Magnesium	1.02 mg
Manganese	.045 mg
Phosphorus	3.94 mg
Potassium	11.6 mg
Selenium	.597 mcg
Sodium	.872 mg
Zinc	.035 mg
Complex Carbohydrates	0 g
Sugars	3.14 g
Mono-Saccharide	.102 g
Di-Saccharide	.025 g
Alcohol	0 g
Caffeine	0 mg
Water	2.02 g

☺ Cinnamon Bon Bons

Calories	37.9
Protein	1.04 g
Carbohydrates	4.44 g
Fat—Total	1.86 g
Saturated Fat	.8 g
Monounsaturated Fat	.279 g
Polyunsaturated Fat	.635 g
Omega 3 Fatty Acid	.104 g
Omega 6 Fatty Acid	.525 g
Cholesterol	.341 mg
Dietary Fiber	.2 g
Total Vitamin A	4.04 RE
A–Retinol	3.48 RE
A–Carotenoid	.331 RE
Thiamin–B1	.016 mg
Riboflavin–B2	.009 mg
Niacin–B3	.151 mg
Niacin Equivalent	.151 mg
Vitamin B6	.036 mg
Vitamin B12	.004 mcg
Folate	2.03 mcg
Pantothenic	.073 mg
Vitamin C	.817 mg
Vitamin D	.032 mcg
Vitamin E-Alpha E	.067 mg

Calcium	29.3 mg
Copper	.038 mg
Iron	.106 mg
Magnesium	5 mg
Manganese	.058 mg
Phosphorus	12 mg
Potassium	52.7 mg
Selenium	.193 mcg
Sodium	2.5 mg
Zinc	.083 mg
Complex Carbohydrates	1.93 g
Sugars	1.54 g
Mono-Saccharide	0 g
Di-Saccharide	.213 g
Alcohol	0 g
Caffeine	0 mg
Water	9.26 g

☉ Citrus Candy

Calories	3.33
Protein	.061 g
Carbohydrates	1 g
Fat—Total	.008 g
Saturated Fat	.001 g
Monounsaturated Fat	.001 g
Polyunsaturated Fat	.001 g
Omega 3 Fatty Acid	.001 g
Omega 6 Fatty Acid	.001 g
Cholesterol	0 mg
Dietary Fiber	.136 g
Total Vitamin A	1.68 RE
A–Retinol	0 RE
A–Carotenoid	1.68 RE
Thiamin–B1	.005 mg
Riboflavin–B2	.003 mg
Niacin–B3	.036 mg
Niacin Equivalent	0 mg
Vitamin B6	.007 mg
Vitamin B12	0 mcg
Folate	1.2 mcg
Pantothenic	.019 mg
Vitamin C	5.44 mg
Vitamin D	0 mcg
Vitamin E-Alpha E	.016 mg

Calcium	6.44 mg
Copper	.003 mg
Iron	.032 mg
Magnesium	.88 mg
Manganese	0 mg
Phosphorus	.84 mg
Potassium	8.47 mg
Selenium	.003 mcg
Sodium	.12 mg
Zinc	.01 mg
Complex Carbohydrates	.867 g
Sugars	0 g
Mono-Saccharide	0 g
Di-Saccharide	0 g
Alcohol	0 g
Caffeine	0 mg
Water	2.9 g

◉ Coated Citrus Candy

Calories	19.2
Protein	.586 g
Carbohydrates	2.47 g
Fat—Total	.835 g
Saturated Fat	.731 g
Monounsaturated Fat	.001 g
Polyunsaturated Fat	.001 g
Omega 3 Fatty Acid	0 g
Omega 6 Fatty Acid	.001 g
Cholesterol	.302 mg
Dietary Fiber	.054 g
Total Vitamin A	.915 RE
A–Retinol	0 RE
A–Carotenoid	.672 RE
Thiamin–B1	.002 mg
Riboflavin–B2	.001 mg
Niacin–B3	.014 mg
Niacin Equivalent	0 mg
Vitamin B6	.003 mg
Vitamin B12	0 mcg
Folate	.48 mcg
Pantothenic	.008 mg
Vitamin C	2.18 mg
Vitamin D	0 mcg
Vitamin E-Alpha E	.006 mg

Calcium	26.5 mg
Copper	.001 mg
Iron	.047 mg
Magnesium	.352 mg
Manganese	0 mg
Phosphorus	.336 mg
Potassium	3.39 mg
Selenium	.001 mcg
Sodium	.048 mg
Zinc	.004 mg
Complex Carbohydrates	.347 g
Sugars	1.3 g
Mono-Saccharide	0 g
Di-Saccharide	0 g
Alcohol	0 g
Caffeine	0 mg
Water	1.16 g

⊚ Cocoa Balls

Calories	19.5
Protein	.453 g
Carbohydrates	1.87 g
Fat—Total	1.37 g
Saturated Fat	.268 g
Monounsaturated Fat	.759 g
Polyunsaturated Fat	.276 g
Omega 3 Fatty Acid	.013 g
Omega 6 Fatty Acid	.262 g
Cholesterol	.693 mg
Dietary Fiber	.36 g
Total Vitamin A	1.87 RE
A–Retinol	1.49 RE
A–Carotenoid	.383 RE
Thiamin–B1	.016 mg
Riboflavin–B2	.013 mg
Niacin–B3	.037 mg
Niacin Equivalent	.037 mg
Vitamin B6	.005 mg
Vitamin B12	.009 mcg
Folate	1.13 mcg
Pantothenic	.045 mg
Vitamin C	.085 mg
Vitamin D	.002 mcg
Vitamin E-Alpha E	.053 mg

Calcium	7.47 mg
Copper	.052 mg
Iron	.158 mg
Magnesium	6.84 mg
Manganese	.105 mg
Phosphorus	16.1 mg
Potassium	26.9 mg
Selenium	.28 mcg
Sodium	2.79 mg
Zinc	.165 mg
Complex Carbohydrates	.312 g
Sugars	1.2 g
Mono-Saccharide	.005 g
Di-Saccharide	1.17 g
Alcohol	0 g
Caffeine	1.98 mg
Water	.761 g

⊚ Coconut Crisps

Calories	8.4
Protein	.134 g
Carbohydrates	.401 g
Fat—Total	.738 g
Saturated Fat	.637 g
Monounsaturated Fat	.048 g
Polyunsaturated Fat	.01 g
Omega 3 Fatty Acid	.001 g
Omega 6 Fatty Acid	.009 g
Cholesterol	.277 mg
Dietary Fiber	.188 g
Total Vitamin A	.63 RE
A–Retinol	.549 RE
A–Carotenoid	.061 RE
Thiamin–B1	.002 mg
Riboflavin–B2	.004 mg
Niacin–B3	.013 mg
Niacin Equivalent	.013 mg
Vitamin B6	.002 mg
Vitamin B12	.007 mcg
Folate	.629 mcg
Pantothenic	.012 mg
Vitamin C	.085 mg
Vitamin D	.02 mcg
Vitamin E-Alpha E	.016 mg

Calcium	2.7 mg
Copper	.009 mg
Iron	.05 mg
Magnesium	.913 mg
Manganese	.03 mg
Phosphorus	4.16 mg
Potassium	10.2 mg
Selenium	.436 mcg
Sodium	1.4 mg
Zinc	.03 mg
Complex Carbohydrates	0 g
Sugars	.22 g
Mono-Saccharide	.068 g
Di-Saccharide	.097 g
Alcohol	0 g
Caffeine	0 mg
Water	2.75 g

⊚ Coconut Delight

Calories	22.4
Protein	.523 g
Carbohydrates	1.74 g
Fat—Total	1.57 g
Saturated Fat	1.39 g
Monounsaturated Fat	.046 g
Polyunsaturated Fat	.012 g
Omega 3 Fatty Acid	0 g
Omega 6 Fatty Acid	.012 g
Cholesterol	.181 mg
Dietary Fiber	.301 g
Total Vitamin A	.146 RE
A–Retinol	0 RE
A–Carotenoid	0 RE
Thiamin–B1	.002 mg
Riboflavin–B2	.004 mg
Niacin–B3	.018 mg
Niacin Equivalent	.018 mg
Vitamin B6	.002 mg
Vitamin B12	.002 mcg
Folate	.867 mcg
Pantothenic	.01 mg
Vitamin C	.106 mg
Vitamin D	0 mcg
Vitamin E-Alpha E	.023 mg

Calcium	14.8 mg
Copper	.014 mg
Iron	.099 mg
Magnesium	1.11 mg
Manganese	.048 mg
Phosphorus	3.71 mg
Potassium	12.5 mg
Selenium	.765 mcg
Sodium	1.88 mg
Zinc	.036 mg
Complex Carbohydrates	0 g
Sugars	.986 g
Mono-Saccharide	.117 g
Di-Saccharide	.003 g
Alcohol	0 g
Caffeine	0 mg
Water	2.17 g

⊙ Coconut Drops

Calories	19.2
Protein	.291 g
Carbohydrates	.509 g
Fat—Total	1.87 g
Saturated Fat	1.42 g
Monounsaturated Fat	.295 g
Polyunsaturated Fat	.043 g
Omega 3 Fatty Acid	.013 g
Omega 6 Fatty Acid	.031 g
Cholesterol	2.83 mg
Dietary Fiber	.271 g
Total Vitamin A	11.3 RE
A–Retinol	10.7 RE
A–Carotenoid	.593 RE
Thiamin–B1	.002 mg
Riboflavin–B2	.006 mg
Niacin–B3	.018 mg
Niacin Equivalent	.018 mg
Vitamin B6	.003 mg
Vitamin B12	.011 mcg
Folate	1.1 mcg
Pantothenic	.016 mg
Vitamin C	.096 mg
Vitamin D	.005 mcg
Vitamin E-Alpha E	.045 mg

Calcium	2.46 mg
Copper	.013 mg
Iron	.101 mg
Magnesium	1.09 mg
Manganese	.043 mg
Phosphorus	5.94 mg
Potassium	13.4 mg
Selenium	.633 mcg
Sodium	8.21 mg
Zinc	.046 mg
Complex Carbohydrates	0 g
Sugars	.248 g
Mono-Saccharide	.098 g
Di-Saccharide	.047 g
Alcohol	0 g
Caffeine	0 mg
Water	2.74 g

⊚ Coconut Rolls

Calories	10.9
Protein	.038 g
Carbohydrates	.086 g
Fat—Total	1.18 g
Saturated Fat	.433 g
Monounsaturated Fat	.443 g
Polyunsaturated Fat	.247 g
Omega 3 Fatty Acid	.006 g
Omega 6 Fatty Acid	.241 g
Cholesterol	1.1 mg
Dietary Fiber	.031 g
Total Vitamin A	12.3 RE
A–Retinol	11.3 RE
A–Carotenoid	.983 RE
Thiamin–B1	.001 mg
Riboflavin–B2	.002 mg
Niacin–B3	.002 mg
Niacin Equivalent	.002 mg
Vitamin B6	.001 mg
Vitamin B12	.002 mcg
Folate	.131 mcg
Pantothenic	.004 mg
Vitamin C	.018 mg
Vitamin D	.002 mcg
Vitamin E-Alpha E	.132 mg

Calcium	.903 mg
Copper	.002 mg
Iron	.008 mg
Magnesium	.193 mg
Manganese	.005 mg
Phosphorus	1.11 mg
Potassium	2.38 mg
Selenium	.072 mcg
Sodium	.43 mg
Zinc	.006 mg
Complex Carbohydrates	0 g
Sugars	.056 g
Mono-Saccharide	.011 g
Di-Saccharide	.03 g
Alcohol	0 g
Caffeine	0 mg
Water	.986 g

⑨ Coconut Sticks

Calories	51.6
Protein	1.03 g
Carbohydrates	8.21 g
Fat—Total	2.17 g
Saturated Fat	.486 g
Monounsaturated Fat	1.15 g
Polyunsaturated Fat	.425 g
Omega 3 Fatty Acid	.012 g
Omega 6 Fatty Acid	.41 g
Cholesterol	0 mg
Dietary Fiber	1.46 g
Total Vitamin A	1.51 RE
A–Retinol	0 RE
A–Carotenoid	1.51 RE
Thiamin–B1	.016 mg
Riboflavin–B2	.035 mg
Niacin–B3	.193 mg
Niacin Equivalent	.194 mg
Vitamin B6	.03 mg
Vitamin B12	0 mcg
Folate	3.02 mcg
Pantothenic	.068 mg
Vitamin C	.144 mg
Vitamin D	0 mcg
Vitamin E-Alpha E	.817 mg

Calcium	25.1 mg
Copper	.07 mg
Iron	.398 mg
Magnesium	16.6 mg
Manganese	.133 mg
Phosphorus	25.7 mg
Potassium	108 mg
Selenium	1.03 mcg
Sodium	1.81 mg
Zinc	.164 mg
Complex Carbohydrates	.172 g
Sugars	6.61 g
Mono-Saccharide	6.7 g
Di-Saccharide	.91 g
Alcohol	0 g
Caffeine	0 mg
Water	3.83 g

⑨ Cranberry Banana Loaf Cake

Calories	64.4
Protein	1.28 g
Carbohydrates	9.73 g
Fat—Total	2.43 g
Saturated Fat	.29 g
Monounsaturated Fat	.5 g
Polyunsaturated Fat	1.54 g
Omega 3 Fatty Acid	.077 g
Omega 6 Fatty Acid	1.45 g
Cholesterol	0 mg
Dietary Fiber	.659 g
Total Vitamin A	1.34 RE
A–Retinol	0 RE
A–Carotenoid	1.34 RE
Thiamin–B1	.072 mg
Riboflavin–B2	.063 mg
Niacin–B3	.551 mg
Niacin Equivalent	.549 mg
Vitamin B6	.091 mg
Vitamin B12	.004 mcg
Folate	5.43 mcg
Pantothenic	.084 mg
Vitamin C	1.61 mg
Vitamin D	0 mcg
Vitamin E-Alpha E	1.11 mg

Calcium	3.16 mg
Copper	.04 mg
Iron	.435 mg
Magnesium	7.69 mg
Manganese	.106 mg
Phosphorus	14.6 mg
Potassium	72.9 mg
Selenium	3.15 mcg
Sodium	3.32 mg
Zinc	.106 mg
Complex Carbohydrates	6.08 g
Sugars	2.96 g
Mono-Saccharide	1.16 g
Di-Saccharide	1.51 g
Alcohol	0 g
Caffeine	0 mg
Water	14.9 g

❂ Cranberry Loaf Cake

Calories	56
Protein	1.06 g
Carbohydrates	7.66 g
Fat—Total	2.46 g
Saturated Fat	.285 g
Monounsaturated Fat	.759 g
Polyunsaturated Fat	1.32 g
Omega 3 Fatty Acid	.016 g
Omega 6 Fatty Acid	1.3 g
Cholesterol	0 mg
Dietary Fiber	.804 g
Total Vitamin A	339 RE
A–Retinol	0 RE
A–Carotenoid	339 RE
Thiamin–B1	.074 mg
Riboflavin–B2	.049 mg
Niacin–B3	.528 mg
Niacin Equivalent	.526 mg
Vitamin B6	.015 mg
Vitamin B12	0 mcg
Folate	4.32 mcg
Pantothenic	.116 mg
Vitamin C	.965 mg
Vitamin D	0 mcg
Vitamin E-Alpha E	1.24 mg

Calcium	5.67 mg
Copper	.04 mg
Iron	.601 mg
Magnesium	6.56 mg
Manganese	.122 mg
Phosphorus	16.7 mg
Potassium	45.2 mg
Selenium	2.91 mcg
Sodium	.957 mg
Zinc	.135 mg
Complex Carbohydrates	5.96 g
Sugars	.87 g
Mono-Saccharide	.071 g
Di-Saccharide	.068 g
Alcohol	0 g
Caffeine	0 mg
Water	16.7 g

◉ Cream Delight

Calories	25.8
Protein	.723 g
Carbohydrates	2.62 g
Fat—Total	1.41 g
Saturated Fat	1.14 g
Monounsaturated Fat	.106 g
Polyunsaturated Fat	.014 g
Omega 3 Fatty Acid	.005 g
Omega 6 Fatty Acid	.008 g
Cholesterol	1.74 mg
Dietary Fiber	0 g
Total Vitamin A	4.47 RE
A–Retinol	4.05 RE
A–Carotenoid	.119 RE
Thiamin–B1	0 mg
Riboflavin–B2	.001 mg
Niacin–B3	0 mg
Niacin Equivalent	0 mg
Vitamin B6	0 mg
Vitamin B12	.002 mcg
Folate	.037 mcg
Pantothenic	.003 mg
Vitamin C	.006 mg
Vitamin D	.013 mcg
Vitamin E-Alpha E	.01 mg

Calcium	30.5 mg
Copper	0 mg
Iron	.043 mg
Magnesium	.07 mg
Manganese	0 mg
Phosphorus	.621 mg
Potassium	.746 mg
Selenium	.006 mcg
Sodium	.373 mg
Zinc	.002 mg
Complex Carbohydrates	0 g
Sugars	1.65 g
Mono-Saccharide	0 g
Di-Saccharide	.028 g
Alcohol	0 g
Caffeine	0 mg
Water	.572 g

☺ Creamy Fudge

Calories	19.1
Protein	.797 g
Carbohydrates	.668 g
Fat—Total	1.59 g
Saturated Fat	.152 g
Monounsaturated Fat	1.03 g
Polyunsaturated Fat	.335 g
Omega 3 Fatty Acid	.011 g
Omega 6 Fatty Acid	.321 g
Cholesterol	.234 mg
Dietary Fiber	.291 g
Total Vitamin A	3.73 RE
A–Retinol	0 RE
A–Carotenoid	0 RE
Thiamin–B1	.006 mg
Riboflavin–B2	.026 mg
Niacin–B3	.102 mg
Niacin Equivalent	.103 mg
Vitamin B6	.003 mg
Vitamin B12	0 mcg
Folate	1.79 mcg
Pantothenic	.014 mg
Vitamin C	.018 mg
Vitamin D	0 mcg
Vitamin E-Alpha E	.731 mg

Calcium	8.11 mg
Copper	.029 mg
Iron	.112 mg
Magnesium	9.02 mg
Manganese	.069 mg
Phosphorus	15.8 mg
Potassium	22.3 mg
Selenium	.143 mcg
Sodium	8.3 mg
Zinc	.089 mg
Complex Carbohydrates	.161 g
Sugars	.171 g
Mono-Saccharide	0 g
Di-Saccharide	.158 g
Alcohol	0 g
Caffeine	0 mg
Water	.135 g

☺ Creamy Strawberries

Calories	58.7
Protein	2.31 g
Carbohydrates	6.66 g
Fat—Total	2.51 g
Saturated Fat	2.19 g
Monounsaturated Fat	.002 g
Polyunsaturated Fat	.008 g
Omega 3 Fatty Acid	.003 g
Omega 6 Fatty Acid	.004 g
Cholesterol	1.66 mg
Dietary Fiber	.064 g
Total Vitamin A	12.8 RE
A–Retinol	0 RE
A–Carotenoid	.124 RE
Thiamin–B1	.001 mg
Riboflavin–B2	.011 mg
Niacin–B3	.01 mg
Niacin Equivalent	.01 mg
Vitamin B6	.002 mg
Vitamin B12	0 mcg
Folate	.735 mcg
Pantothenic	.014 mg
Vitamin C	2.35 mg
Vitamin D	0 mcg
Vitamin E-Alpha E	.006 mg

Calcium	72.3 mg
Copper	.002 mg
Iron	.119 mg
Magnesium	.415 mg
Manganese	.012 mg
Phosphorus	.788 mg
Potassium	6.9 mg
Selenium	.037 mcg
Sodium	25.5 mg
Zinc	.005 mg
Complex Carbohydrates	0 g
Sugars	4.13 g
Mono-Saccharide	.195 g
Di-Saccharide	.046 g
Alcohol	0 g
Caffeine	0 mg
Water	3.8 g

⊚ Crunch Bars

Calories	80.1
Protein	2.31 g
Carbohydrates	10.3 g
Fat—Total	3.33 g
Saturated Fat	2.54 g
Monounsaturated Fat	.306 g
Polyunsaturated Fat	.088 g
Omega 3 Fatty Acid	.002 g
Omega 6 Fatty Acid	.085 g
Cholesterol	1.01 mg
Dietary Fiber	.128 g
Total Vitamin A	.811 RE
A–Retinol	0 RE
A–Carotenoid	0 RE
Thiamin–B1	.027 mg
Riboflavin–B2	.022 mg
Niacin–B3	.248 mg
Niacin Equivalent	.248 mg
Vitamin B6	.002 mg
Vitamin B12	0 mcg
Folate	1.46 mcg
Pantothenic	.021 mg
Vitamin C	0 mg
Vitamin D	0 mcg
Vitamin E-Alpha E	.025 mg

Calcium	85.4 mg
Copper	.009 mg
Iron	.37 mg
Magnesium	1.28 mg
Manganese	.033 mg
Phosphorus	4.98 mg
Potassium	34.3 mg
Selenium	.554 mcg
Sodium	30.1 mg
Zinc	.037 mg
Complex Carbohydrates	3.18 g
Sugars	4.41 g
Mono-Saccharide	0 g
Di-Saccharide	0 g
Alcohol	0 g
Caffeine	0 mg
Water	.194 g

◎ Crunchy Chocolate Cupcakes

Calories	96.7
Protein	3.3 g
Carbohydrates	13.5 g
Fat—Total	3.4 g
Saturated Fat	2.05 g
Monounsaturated Fat	.398 g
Polyunsaturated Fat	.606 g
Omega 3 Fatty Acid	.029 g
Omega 6 Fatty Acid	.578 g
Cholesterol	.94 mg
Dietary Fiber	.721 g
Total Vitamin A	30.3 RE
A–Retinol	27.7 RE
A–Carotenoid	1.93 RE
Thiamin–B1	.124 mg
Riboflavin–B2	.069 mg
Niacin–B3	.683 mg
Niacin Equivalent	.684 mg
Vitamin B6	.048 mg
Vitamin B12	.04 mcg
Folate	11.4 mcg
Pantothenic	.14 mg
Vitamin C	.102 mg
Vitamin D	.354 mcg
Vitamin E-Alpha E	.739 mg

Calcium	98.4 mg
Copper	.037 mg
Iron	.693 mg
Magnesium	10.5 mg
Manganese	.471 mg
Phosphorus	82.2 mg
Potassium	108 mg
Selenium	5.34 mcg
Sodium	14.6 mg
Zinc	.484 mg
Complex Carbohydrates	6.59 g
Sugars	4.27 g
Mono-Saccharide	.071 g
Di-Saccharide	.761 g
Alcohol	0 g
Caffeine	0 mg
Water	12 g

⑨ Custard Tarts

Calories	56.9
Protein	1.52 g
Carbohydrates	7.63 g
Fat—Total	2.27 g
Saturated Fat	.54 g
Monounsaturated Fat	.806 g
Polyunsaturated Fat	.728 g
Omega 3 Fatty Acid	.017 g
Omega 6 Fatty Acid	.713 g
Cholesterol	22.1 mg
Dietary Fiber	.355 g
Total Vitamin A	49.4 RE
A–Retinol	45.6 RE
A–Carotenoid	3.65 RE
Thiamin–B1	.056 mg
Riboflavin–B2	.07 mg
Niacin–B3	.388 mg
Niacin Equivalent	.389 mg
Vitamin B6	.02 mg
Vitamin B12	.074 mcg
Folate	4.54 mcg
Pantothenic	.123 mg
Vitamin C	.528 mg
Vitamin D	.529 mcg
Vitamin E-Alpha E	.35 mg

Calcium	12.5 mg
Copper	.015 mg
Iron	.41 mg
Magnesium	3.7 mg
Manganese	.055 mg
Phosphorus	23.2 mg
Potassium	46.7 mg
Selenium	3.82 mcg
Sodium	23.6 mg
Zinc	.13 mg
Complex Carbohydrates	4.46 g
Sugars	2.67 g
Mono-Saccharide	.693 g
Di-Saccharide	.49 g
Alcohol	0 g
Caffeine	0 mg
Water	19.9 g

☉ Date Balls

Calories	27.5
Protein	.41 g
Carbohydrates	2.7 g
Fat—Total	1.83 g
Saturated Fat	.506 g
Monounsaturated Fat	.474 g
Polyunsaturated Fat	.743 g
Omega 3 Fatty Acid	.105 g
Omega 6 Fatty Acid	.629 g
Cholesterol	5.33 mg
Dietary Fiber	.338 g
Total Vitamin A	8.01 RE
A–Retinol	7.26 RE
A–Carotenoid	.733 RE
Thiamin–B1	.012 mg
Riboflavin–B2	.008 mg
Niacin–B3	.12 mg
Niacin Equivalent	.12 mg
Vitamin B6	.016 mg
Vitamin B12	.015 mcg
Folate	2.22 mcg
Pantothenic	.049 mg
Vitamin C	.11 mg
Vitamin D	.04 mcg
Vitamin E-Alpha E	.13 mg

Calcium	3.05 mg
Copper	.033 mg
Iron	.119 mg
Magnesium	3.98 mg
Manganese	.075 mg
Phosphorus	9.63 mg
Potassium	26.8 mg
Selenium	.61 mcg
Sodium	5.76 mg
Zinc	.083 mg
Complex Carbohydrates	.725 g
Sugars	1.63 g
Mono-Saccharide	.05 g
Di-Saccharide	1.08 g
Alcohol	0 g
Caffeine	0 mg
Water	1.38 g

⑨ Date Cupcakes

Calories	72.1
Protein	1.51 g
Carbohydrates	11.9 g
Fat—Total	2.17 g
Saturated Fat	.392 g
Monounsaturated Fat	.782 g
Polyunsaturated Fat	.844 g
Omega 3 Fatty Acid	.014 g
Omega 6 Fatty Acid	.832 g
Cholesterol	8.88 mg
Dietary Fiber	.712 g
Total Vitamin A	52.5 RE
A–Retinol	47 RE
A–Carotenoid	5.35 RE
Thiamin–B1	.095 mg
Riboflavin–B2	.069 mg
Niacin–B3	.722 mg
Niacin Equivalent	.721 mg
Vitamin B6	.02 mg
Vitamin B12	.023 mcg
Folate	7.72 mcg
Pantothenic	.122 mg
Vitamin C	4.38 mg
Vitamin D	.53 mcg
Vitamin E-Alpha E	.366 mg

Calcium	14.7 mg
Copper	.03 mg
Iron	.582 mg
Magnesium	4.88 mg
Manganese	.085 mg
Phosphorus	30.8 mg
Potassium	74.6 mg
Selenium	4.29 mcg
Sodium	19.8 mg
Zinc	.114 mg
Complex Carbohydrates	7.54 g
Sugars	3.59 g
Mono-Saccharide	.822 g
Di-Saccharide	1.91 g
Alcohol	0 g
Caffeine	0 mg
Water	14.6 g

⊚ Date Roll

Calories	34.7
Protein	.427 g
Carbohydrates	2.66 g
Fat—Total	2.72 g
Saturated Fat	1.03 g
Monounsaturated Fat	.712 g
Polyunsaturated Fat	.837 g
Omega 3 Fatty Acid	.158 g
Omega 6 Fatty Acid	.67 g
Cholesterol	5.43 mg
Dietary Fiber	.314 g
Total Vitamin A	17.1 RE
A–Retinol	16.2 RE
A–Carotenoid	.873 RE
Thiamin–B1	.011 mg
Riboflavin–B2	.01 mg
Niacin–B3	.088 mg
Niacin Equivalent	.088 mg
Vitamin B6	.018 mg
Vitamin B12	.007 mcg
Folate	1.84 mcg
Pantothenic	.046 mg
Vitamin C	.087 mg
Vitamin D	.052 mcg
Vitamin E-Alpha E	.095 mg

Calcium	5.4 mg
Copper	.037 mg
Iron	.085 mg
Magnesium	4.7 mg
Manganese	.067 mg
Phosphorus	10 mg
Potassium	32.4 mg
Selenium	.18 mcg
Sodium	1.78 mg
Zinc	.073 mg
Complex Carbohydrates	.233 g
Sugars	2.1 g
Mono-Saccharide	0 g
Di-Saccharide	1.48 g
Alcohol	0 g
Caffeine	0 mg
Water	3.03 g

⑨ Dipped Pecans

Calories	55.3
Protein	1.13 g
Carbohydrates	3.62 g
Fat—Total	4.21 g
Saturated Fat	1.46 g
Monounsaturated Fat	1.66 g
Polyunsaturated Fat	.805 g
Omega 3 Fatty Acid	.023 g
Omega 6 Fatty Acid	.784 g
Cholesterol	.454 mg
Dietary Fiber	.125 g
Total Vitamin A	14.8 RE
A–Retinol	12.9 RE
A–Carotenoid	1.51 RE
Thiamin–B1	.023 mg
Riboflavin B2	.007 mg
Niacin–B3	.025 mg
Niacin Equivalent	.025 mg
Vitamin B6	.005 mg
Vitamin B12	.002 mcg
Folate	1.09 mcg
Pantothenic	.048 mg
Vitamin C	.056 mg
Vitamin D	0 mcg
Vitamin E-Alpha E	.266 mg

Calcium	37.1 mg
Copper	.032 mg
Iron	.109 mg
Magnesium	3.55 mg
Manganese	.122 mg
Phosphorus	8.13 mg
Potassium	11.9 mg
Selenium	.265 mcg
Sodium	1.22 mg
Zinc	.148 mg
Complex Carbohydrates	.25 g
Sugars	2.08 g
Mono-Saccharide	.007 g
Di-Saccharide	.108 g
Alcohol	0 g
Caffeine	0 mg
Water	1.02 g

⊚ Dream Balls

Calories	25
Protein	.381 g
Carbohydrates	3.59 g
Fat—Total	1.26 g
Saturated Fat	.123 g
Monounsaturated Fat	.289 g
Polyunsaturated Fat	.784 g
Omega 3 Fatty Acid	.137 g
Omega 6 Fatty Acid	.638 g
Cholesterol	0 mg
Dietary Fiber	.414 g
Total Vitamin A	.589 RE
A–Retinol	0 RE
A–Carotenoid	.589 RE
Thiamin–B1	.012 mg
Riboflavin–B2	.009 mg
Niacin–B3	.114 mg
Niacin Equivalent	.114 mg
Vitamin B6	.029 mg
Vitamin B12	0 mcg
Folate	2.16 mcg
Pantothenic	.047 mg
Vitamin C	.237 mg
Vitamin D	0 mcg
Vitamin E-Alpha E	.061 mg

Calcium	3.21 mg
Copper	.041 mg
Iron	.099 mg
Magnesium	5.26 mg
Manganese	.072 mg
Phosphorus	8.22 mg
Potassium	42.2 mg
Selenium	.191 mcg
Sodium	.332 mg
Zinc	.069 mg
Complex Carbohydrates	.288 g
Sugars	2.88 g
Mono-Saccharide	.144 g
Di-Saccharide	1.93 g
Alcohol	0 g
Caffeine	0 mg
Water	2.33 g

⊚ English Toffee

Calories	57.9
Protein	.942 g
Carbohydrates	1.52 g
Fat—Total	5.58 g
Saturated Fat	1.09 g
Monounsaturated Fat	2.77 g
Polyunsaturated Fat	1.46 g
Omega 3 Fatty Acid	.026 g
Omega 6 Fatty Acid	1.43 g
Cholesterol	.113 mg
Dietary Fiber	.338 g
Total Vitamin A	42.4 RE
A–Retinol	38.7 RE
A–Carotenoid	3.48 RE
Thiamin–B1	.008 mg
Riboflavin–B2	.029 mg
Niacin–B3	.12 mg
Niacin Equivalent	.12 mg
Vitamin B6	.004 mg
Vitamin B12	.002 mcg
Folate	2.11 mcg
Pantothenic	.019 mg
Vitamin C	.025 mg
Vitamin D	0 mcg
Vitamin E-Alpha E	1.4 mg

Calcium	19.2 mg
Copper	.034 mg
Iron	.143 mg
Magnesium	10.6 mg
Manganese	.08 mg
Phosphorus	19 mg
Potassium	27 mg
Selenium	.167 mcg
Sodium	.484 mg
Zinc	.104 mg
Complex Carbohydrates	.188 g
Sugars	.708 g
Mono-Saccharide	0 g
Di-Saccharide	.185 g
Alcohol	0 g
Caffeine	0 mg
Water	.945 g

⊚ Fancy Pecans

Calories	34.2
Protein	.381 g
Carbohydrates	6.53 g
Fat—Total	1.11 g
Saturated Fat	.101 g
Monounsaturated Fat	.656 g
Polyunsaturated Fat	.288 g
Omega 3 Fatty Acid	.011 g
Omega 6 Fatty Acid	.278 g
Cholesterol	0 mg
Dietary Fiber	.799 g
Total Vitamin Λ	1.09 RE
A–Retinol	0 RE
A–Carotenoid	1.09 RE
Thiamin–B1	.021 mg
Riboflavin–B2	.01 mg
Niacin–B3	.101 mg
Niacin Equivalent	.101 mg
Vitamin B6	.023 mg
Vitamin B12	0 mcg
Folate	1.29 mcg
Pantothenic	.065 mg
Vitamin C	.129 mg
Vitamin D	0 mcg
Vitamin E-Alpha E	.075 mg

Calcium	10.5 mg
Copper	.046 mg
Iron	.217 mg
Magnesium	6.52 mg
Manganese	.101 mg
Phosphorus	10.6 mg
Potassium	70.2 mg
Selenium	.571 mcg
Sodium	.908 mg
Zinc	.122 mg
Complex Carbohydrates	.14 g
Sugars	5.6 g
Mono-Saccharide	4.54 g
Di-Saccharide	1.13 g
Alcohol	0 g
Caffeine	0 mg
Water	2.36 g

✿ Fig Sticks

Calories	59.1
Protein	1.49 g
Carbohydrates	8.24 g
Fat—Total	2.86 g
Saturated Fat	.332 g
Monounsaturated Fat	1.52 g
Polyunsaturated Fat	.871 g
Omega 3 Fatty Acid	.02 g
Omega 6 Fatty Acid	.849 g
Cholesterol	0 mg
Dietary Fiber	1.54 g
Total Vitamin A	1.63 RE
A–Retinol	0 RE
A–Carotenoid	1.63 RE
Thiamin–B1	.028 mg
Riboflavin–B2	.037 mg
Niacin–B3	.276 mg
Niacin Equivalent	.276 mg
Vitamin B6	.032 mg
Vitamin B12	0 mcg
Folate	4.56 mcg
Pantothenic	.077 mg
Vitamin C	.11 mg
Vitamin D	0 mcg
Vitamin E-Alpha E	.856 mg

Calcium	27.4 mg
Copper	.093 mg
Iron	.52 mg
Magnesium	22.8 mg
Manganese	.145 mg
Phosphorus	39.2 mg
Potassium	112 mg
Selenium	.982 mcg
Sodium	2.36 mg
Zinc	.347 mg
Complex Carbohydrates	.199 g
Sugars	6.57 g
Mono-Saccharide	6.67 g
Di-Saccharide	.909 g
Alcohol	0 g
Caffeine	0 mg
Water	3.46 g

⊚ Filled Fruit

Calories	53.1
Protein	1.39 g
Carbohydrates	3.15 g
Fat—Total	3.9 g
Saturated Fat	.717 g
Monounsaturated Fat	1.78 g
Polyunsaturated Fat	1.2 g
Omega 3 Fatty Acid	.014 g
Omega 6 Fatty Acid	1.19 g
Cholesterol	1.25 mg
Dietary Fiber	.465 g
Total Vitamin A	134 RE
A–Retinol	43 RE
A–Carotenoid	71.4 RE
Thiamin–B1	.008 mg
Riboflavin–B2	.026 mg
Niacin–B3	.156 mg
Niacin Equivalent	.156 mg
Vitamin B6	.014 mg
Vitamin B12	.003 mcg
Folate	2.25 mcg
Pantothenic	.064 mg
Vitamin C	2.59 mg
Vitamin D	0 mcg
Vitamin E-Alpha E	.837 mg

Calcium	4.47 mg
Copper	.023 mg
Iron	.14 mg
Magnesium	2.14 mg
Manganese	.02 mg
Phosphorus	5.55 mg
Potassium	77.7 mg
Selenium	.337 mcg
Sodium	42.8 mg
Zinc	.067 mg
Complex Carbohydrates	0 g
Sugars	2.28 g
Mono-Saccharide	.595 g
Di-Saccharide	1.6 g
Alcohol	0 g
Caffeine	0 mg
Water	23.4 g

☉ Friendly Dates

Calories	57.8
Protein	1.09 g
Carbohydrates	5.24 g
Fat—Total	4.14 g
Saturated Fat	.382 g
Monounsaturated Fat	.95 g
Polyunsaturated Fat	2.61 g
Omega 3 Fatty Acid	.451 g
Omega 6 Fatty Acid	2.12 g
Cholesterol	0 mg
Dietary Fiber	.785 g
Total Vitamin A	1.43 RE
A–Retinol	0 RE
A–Carotenoid	1.43 RE
Thiamin–B1	.03 mg
Riboflavin–B2	.015 mg
Niacin–B3	.153 mg
Niacin Equivalent	.151 mg
Vitamin B6	.049 mg
Vitamin B12	0 mcg
Folate	5.06 mcg
Pantothenic	.078 mg
Vitamin C	.74 mg
Vitamin D	0 mcg
Vitamin E-Alpha E	.185 mg

Calcium	11.6 mg
Copper	.109 mg
Iron	.26 mg
Magnesium	13.9 mg
Manganese	.211 mg
Phosphorus	24.1 mg
Potassium	72.9 mg
Selenium	.556 mcg
Sodium	1.07 mg
Zinc	.205 mg
Complex Carbohydrates	.815 g
Sugars	3.64 g
Mono-Saccharide	1.68 g
Di-Saccharide	1.59 g
Alcohol	0 g
Caffeine	0 mg
Water	2.29 g

☺ Frosted Fruit

Calories	3.7
Protein	.203 g
Carbohydrates	.721 g
Fat—Total	.037 g
Saturated Fat	.002 g
Monounsaturated Fat	.005 g
Polyunsaturated Fat	.019 g
Omega 3 Fatty Acid	.008 g
Omega 6 Fatty Acid	.011 g
Cholesterol	0 mg
Dietary Fiber	.154 g
Total Vitamin A	.302 RE
A–Retinol	0 RE
A–Carotenoid	.302 RE
Thiamin–B1	.002 mg
Riboflavin–B2	.013 mg
Niacin–B3	.024 mg
Niacin Equivalent	.024 mg
Vitamin B6	.006 mg
Vitamin B12	.003 mcg
Folate	1.83 mcg
Pantothenic	.036 mg
Vitamin C	5.71 mg
Vitamin D	0 mcg
Vitamin E-Alpha E	.014 mg

Calcium	1.5 mg
Copper	.005 mg
Iron	.039 mg
Magnesium	1.16 mg
Manganese	.029 mg
Phosphorus	2.09 mg
Potassium	18.7 mg
Selenium	.328 mcg
Sodium	2.32 mg
Zinc	.013 mg
Complex Carbohydrates	0 g
Sugars	.582 g
Mono-Saccharide	.488 g
Di-Saccharide	.111 g
Alcohol	0 g
Caffeine	0 mg
Water	10.4 g

⊚ Frozen Fruit

Calories	41
Protein	.79 g
Carbohydrates	6.01 g
Fat—Total	1.75 g
Saturated Fat	1.41 g
Monounsaturated Fat	.144 g
Polyunsaturated Fat	.079 g
Omega 3 Fatty Acid	.025 g
Omega 6 Fatty Acid	.034 g
Cholesterol	.283 mg
Dietary Fiber	.254 g
Total Vitamin A	16.6 RE
A–Retinol	9.2 RE
A–Carotenoid	7.39 RE
Thiamin–B1	.02 mg
Riboflavin–B2	.033 mg
Niacin–B3	.097 mg
Niacin Equivalent	.086 mg
Vitamin B6	.022 mg
Vitamin B12	.019 mcg
Folate	2.81 mcg
Pantothenic	.086 mg
Vitamin C	2.88 mg
Vitamin D	.157 mcg
Vitamin E-Alpha E	.047 mg

Calcium	25.2 mg
Copper	.027 mg
Iron	.113 mg
Magnesium	5.05 mg
Manganese	.289 mg
Phosphorus	17.7 mg
Potassium	52.7 mg
Selenium	.276 mcg
Sodium	11.5 mg
Zinc	.091 mg
Complex Carbohydrates	.205 g
Sugars	5.56 g
Mono-Saccharide	.861 g
Di-Saccharide	1.43 g
Alcohol	0 g
Caffeine	0 mg
Water	30.5 g

☉ Fruit Bars

Calories	66.5
Protein	.968 g
Carbohydrates	10.6 g
Fat—Total	2.92 g
Saturated Fat	.897 g
Monounsaturated Fat	.5 g
Polyunsaturated Fat	1.36 g
Omega 3 Fatty Acid	.156 g
Omega 6 Fatty Acid	1.19 g
Cholesterol	0 mg
Dietary Fiber	1.45 g
Total Vitamin A	1.49 RE
A–Retinol	0 RE
A–Carotenoid	1.49 RE
Thiamin–B1	.026 mg
Riboflavin–B2	.02 mg
Niacin–B3	.25 mg
Niacin Equivalent	.249 mg
Vitamin B6	.053 mg
Vitamin B12	0 mcg
Folate	5.95 mcg
Pantothenic	.167 mg
Vitamin C	.293 mg
Vitamin D	0 mcg
Vitamin E-Alpha E	.764 mg

Calcium	15.5 mg
Copper	.104 mg
Iron	.444 mg
Magnesium	12.4 mg
Manganese	.171 mg
Phosphorus	31.5 mg
Potassium	120 mg
Selenium	2.1 mcg
Sodium	1.95 mg
Zinc	.202 mg
Complex Carbohydrates	.385 g
Sugars	8.75 g
Mono-Saccharide	5.55 g
Di-Saccharide	2.52 g
Alcohol	0 g
Caffeine	0 mg
Water	4.47 g

⑨ Fruit Crêpes

Calories	58.3
Protein	2.32 g
Carbohydrates	8.14 g
Fat—Total	2.1 g
Saturated Fat	.838 g
Monounsaturated Fat	.68 g
Polyunsaturated Fat	.244 g
Omega 3 Fatty Acid	.028 g
Omega 6 Fatty Acid	.216 g
Cholesterol	56 mg
Dietary Fiber	.907 g
Total Vitamin A	32.6 RE
A–Retinol	29.4 RE
A–Carotenoid	3.05 RE
Thiamin–B1	.023 mg
Riboflavin–B2	.103 mg
Niacin–B3	.062 mg
Niacin Equivalent	.062 mg
Vitamin B6	.048 mg
Vitamin B12	.198 mcg
Folate	8.18 mcg
Pantothenic	.249 mg
Vitamin C	2.81 mg
Vitamin D	.366 mcg
Vitamin E-Alpha E	.4 mg

Calcium	33.5 mg
Copper	.023 mg
Iron	.273 mg
Magnesium	6.28 mg
Manganese	.025 mg
Phosphorus	44.5 mg
Potassium	99 mg
Selenium	4.39 mcg
Sodium	25.8 mg
Zinc	.234 mg
Complex Carbohydrates	.005 g
Sugars	6.64 g
Mono-Saccharide	3.99 g
Di-Saccharide	2.15 g
Alcohol	0 g
Caffeine	0 mg
Water	65.9 g

☺ Fruit Surprise

Calories	26.2
Protein	.643 g
Carbohydrates	2.11 g
Fat—Total	1.77 g
Saturated Fat	1.08 g
Monounsaturated Fat	.443 g
Polyunsaturated Fat	.113 g
Omega 3 Fatty Acid	.011 g
Omega 6 Fatty Acid	.101 g
Cholesterol	2.26 mg
Dietary Fiber	.148 g
Total Vitamin A	6.53 RE
A–Retinol	6.08 RE
A–Carotenoid	.274 RE
Thiamin–B1	.003 mg
Riboflavin–B2	.009 mg
Niacin–B3	.039 mg
Niacin Equivalent	.039 mg
Vitamin B6	.003 mg
Vitamin B12	.003 mcg
Folate	.789 mcg
Pantothenic	.01 mg
Vitamin C	.052 mg
Vitamin D	.019 mcg
Vitamin E-Alpha E	.217 mg

Calcium	21.2 mg
Copper	.011 mg
Iron	.072 mg
Magnesium	3.01 mg
Manganese	.028 mg
Phosphorus	5.95 mg
Potassium	13.5 mg
Selenium	.154 mcg
Sodium	.758 mg
Zinc	.035 mg
Complex Carbohydrates	.111 g
Sugars	1.28 g
Mono-Saccharide	.017 g
Di-Saccharide	.084 g
Alcohol	0 g
Caffeine	0 mg
Water	1.14 g

⑨ Graham Cracker Crust

Calories	70.4
Protein	.856 g
Carbohydrates	9.24 g
Fat—Total	3.41 g
Saturated Fat	.666 g
Monounsaturated Fat	1.43 g
Polyunsaturated Fat	1.11 g
Omega 3 Fatty Acid	.019 g
Omega 6 Fatty Acid	1.09 g
Cholesterol	0 mg
Dietary Fiber	.324 g
Total Vitamin A	56.4 RE
A–Retinol	51.6 RE
A–Carotenoid	4.64 RE
Thiamin–B1	.027 mg
Riboflavin–B2	.039 mg
Niacin–B3	.495 mg
Niacin Equivalent	.495 mg
Vitamin B6	.008 mg
Vitamin B12	.003 mcg
Folate	2.08 mcg
Pantothenic	.067 mg
Vitamin C	.006 mg
Vitamin D	.604 mcg
Vitamin E-Alpha E	.424 mg

Calcium	3.89 mg
Copper	.024 mg
Iron	.449 mg
Magnesium	3.69 mg
Manganese	.097 mg
Phosphorus	13.3 mg
Potassium	17.6 mg
Selenium	1.32 mcg
Sodium	92.6 mg
Zinc	.097 mg
Complex Carbohydrates	3.23 g
Sugars	5.68 g
Mono-Saccharide	0 g
Di-Saccharide	0 g
Alcohol	0 g
Caffeine	0 mg
Water	3.83 g

⑨ Granola Candy

Calories	29.9
Protein	.653 g
Carbohydrates	3.5 g
Fat—Total	1.66 g
Saturated Fat	.492 g
Monounsaturated Fat	.403 g
Polyunsaturated Fat	.72 g
Omega 3 Fatty Acid	.034 g
Omega 6 Fatty Acid	.682 g
Cholesterol	0 mg
Dietary Fiber	.612 g
Total Vitamin A	.178 RE
A–Retinol	0 RE
A–Carotenoid	.178 RE
Thiamin–B1	.031 mg
Riboflavin–B2	.013 mg
Niacin–B3	.094 mg
Niacin Equivalent	.094 mg
Vitamin B6	.018 mg
Vitamin B12	0 mcg
Folate	4.34 mcg
Pantothenic	.033 mg
Vitamin C	.078 mg
Vitamin D	0 mcg
Vitamin E-Alpha E	.244 mg

Calcium	3.34 mg
Copper	.033 mg
Iron	.223 mg
Magnesium	6.18 mg
Manganese	.012 mg
Phosphorus	21.7 mg
Potassium	28.5 mg
Selenium	1.18 mcg
Sodium	5.01 mg
Zinc	.196 mg
Complex Carbohydrates	.879 g
Sugars	1.44 g
Mono-Saccharide	.508 g
Di-Saccharide	.909 g
Alcohol	0 g
Caffeine	0 mg
Water	1.61 g

⑨ Granola Delight

Calories	31.3
Protein	.358 g
Carbohydrates	3.97 g
Fat—Total	1.77 g
Saturated Fat	.642 g
Monounsaturated Fat	.527 g
Polyunsaturated Fat	.529 g
Omega 3 Fatty Acid	.016 g
Omega 6 Fatty Acid	.511 g
Cholesterol	0 mg
Dietary Fiber	.562 g
Total Vitamin A	9.62 RE
A–Retinol	8.6 RE
A–Carotenoid	.993 RE
Thiamin–B1	.016 mg
Riboflavin–B2	.009 mg
Niacin–B3	.109 mg
Niacin Equivalent	.109 mg
Vitamin B6	.014 mg
Vitamin B12	.001 mcg
Folate	2.38 mcg
Pantothenic	.04 mg
Vitamin C	.065 mg
Vitamin D	0 mcg
Vitamin E-Alpha E	.229 mg

Calcium	2.62 mg
Copper	.026 mg
Iron	.148 mg
Magnesium	3.85 mg
Manganese	.029 mg
Phosphorus	11.2 mg
Potassium	34.6 mg
Selenium	.726 mcg
Sodium	4.05 mg
Zinc	.098 mg
Complex Carbohydrates	.352 g
Sugars	2.59 g
Mono-Saccharide	.237 g
Di-Saccharide	1.69 g
Alcohol	0 g
Caffeine	0 mg
Water	2.38 g

⊚ Happy Trails

Calories	85.6
Protein	2.59 g
Carbohydrates	9.48 g
Fat—Total	4.38 g
Saturated Fat	2.39 g
Monounsaturated Fat	.756 g
Polyunsaturated Fat	.879 g
Omega 3 Fatty Acid	.029 g
Omega 6 Fatty Acid	.845 g
Cholesterol	.854 mg
Dietary Fiber	.582 g
Total Vitamin A	.837 RE
A–Retinol	0 RE
A–Carotenoid	.151 RE
Thiamin–B1	.037 mg
Riboflavin–B2	.013 mg
Niacin–B3	.378 mg
Niacin Equivalent	.378 mg
Vitamin B6	.021 mg
Vitamin B12	.003 mcg
Folate	6.09 mcg
Pantothenic	.054 mg
Vitamin C	.083 mg
Vitamin D	.035 mcg
Vitamin E-Alpha E	.33 mg

Calcium	71.3 mg
Copper	.038 mg
Iron	.332 mg
Magnesium	8.44 mg
Manganese	.049 mg
Phosphorus	24.7 mg
Potassium	33.8 mg
Selenium	1.14 mcg
Sodium	7.81 mg
Zinc	.231 mg
Complex Carbohydrates	1.69 g
Sugars	5.02 g
Mono-Saccharide	.421 g
Di-Saccharide	.913 g
Alcohol	0 g
Caffeine	0 mg
Water	.224 g

⑨ Haupia

Calories	7.51
Protein	.387 g
Carbohydrates	.228 g
Fat—Total	.607 g
Saturated Fat	.538 g
Monounsaturated Fat	.027 g
Polyunsaturated Fat	.007 g
Omega 3 Fatty Acid	0 g
Omega 6 Fatty Acid	.007 g
Cholesterol	.055 mg
Dietary Fiber	.032 g
Total Vitamin A	1.86 RE
A–Retinol	1.86 RE
A–Carotenoid	0 RE
Thiamin–B1	.002 mg
Riboflavin–B2	.005 mg
Niacin–B3	.021 mg
Niacin Equivalent	.021 mg
Vitamin B6	.002 mg
Vitamin B12	.012 mcg
Folate	.619 mcg
Pantothenic	.015 mg
Vitamin C	.058 mg
Vitamin D	.031 mcg
Vitamin E-Alpha E	.018 mg

Calcium	4.42 mg
Copper	.012 mg
Iron	.098 mg
Magnesium	1.71 mg
Manganese	.022 mg
Phosphorus	5.9 mg
Potassium	11.3 mg
Selenium	.235 mcg
Sodium	2.46 mg
Zinc	.028 mg
Complex Carbohydrates	0 g
Sugars	.197 g
Mono-Saccharide	0 g
Di-Saccharide	.149 g
Alcohol	0 g
Caffeine	0 mg
Water	4.88 g

☺ Heavenly Puffs

Calories	102
Protein	2.51 g
Carbohydrates	16 g
Fat—Total	3.01 g
Saturated Fat	.537 g
Monounsaturated Fat	1.07 g
Polyunsaturated Fat	1.18 g
Omega 3 Fatty Acid	.02 g
Omega 6 Fatty Acid	1.16 g
Cholesterol	12.2 mg
Dietary Fiber	.743 g
Total Vitamin A	69.9 RE
A–Retinol	64.4 RE
A–Carotenoid	5.34 RE
Thiamin–B1	.163 mg
Riboflavin–B2	.118 mg
Niacin–B3	1.22 mg
Niacin Equivalent	1.22 mg
Vitamin B6	.015 mg
Vitamin B12	.032 mcg
Folate	6.73 mcg
Pantothenic	.129 mg
Vitamin C	.043 mg
Vitamin D	.727 mcg
Vitamin E-Alpha E	.504 mg

Calcium	7.25 mg
Copper	.031 mg
Iron	1.05 mg
Magnesium	4.98 mg
Manganese	.163 mg
Phosphorus	28.2 mg
Potassium	59.2 mg
Selenium	7.87 mcg
Sodium	62.9 mg
Zinc	.179 mg
Complex Carbohydrates	14.8 g
Sugars	.428 g
Mono-Saccharide	.221 g
Di-Saccharide	.082 g
Alcohol	0 g
Caffeine	0 mg
Water	8.38 g

✆ Lemon Biscotti

Calories	69.3
Protein	2.03 g
Carbohydrates	6.88 g
Fat—Total	4.2 g
Saturated Fat	.681 g
Monounsaturated Fat	1.79 g
Polyunsaturated Fat	1.47 g
Omega 3 Fatty Acid	.041 g
Omega 6 Fatty Acid	1.43 g
Cholesterol	13.1 mg
Dietary Fiber	.836 g
Total Vitamin A	25.2 RE
A–Retinol	23.1 RE
A–Carotenoid	2.04 RE
Thiamin–B1	.12 mg
Riboflavin–B2	.068 mg
Niacin–B3	.617 mg
Niacin Equivalent	.617 mg
Vitamin B6	.016 mg
Vitamin B12	.034 mcg
Folate	6.56 mcg
Pantothenic	.101 mg
Vitamin C	.451 mg
Vitamin D	.241 mcg
Vitamin E-Alpha E	.388 mg

Calcium	15 mg
Copper	.07 mg
Iron	.627 mg
Magnesium	13.5 mg
Manganese	.221 mg
Phosphorus	37.9 mg
Potassium	76.7 mg
Selenium	3.77 mcg
Sodium	15.4 mg
Zinc	.272 mg
Complex Carbohydrates	5.6 g
Sugars	.437 g
Mono-Saccharide	.119 g
Di-Saccharide	.053 g
Alcohol	0 g
Caffeine	0 mg
Water	5.68 g

◎ Lemon Cheesecake

Calories	121
Protein	4.73 g
Carbohydrates	17.9 g
Fat—Total	3.54 g
Saturated Fat	.731 g
Monounsaturated Fat	1.46 g
Polyunsaturated Fat	1.12 g
Omega 3 Fatty Acid	.021 g
Omega 6 Fatty Acid	1.1 g
Cholesterol	1.84 mg
Dietary Fiber	.364 g
Total Vitamin A	116 RE
A–Retinol	111 RE
A–Carotenoid	4.68 RE
Thiamin–B1	.051 mg
Riboflavin–B2	.197 mg
Niacin–B3	.585 mg
Niacin Equivalent	.585 mg
Vitamin B6	.037 mg
Vitamin B12	.125 mcg
Folate	6.61 mcg
Pantothenic	.446 mg
Vitamin C	1.39 mg
Vitamin D	1.62 mcg
Vitamin E-Alpha E	.43 mg

Calcium	152 mg
Copper	.033 mg
Iron	.608 mg
Magnesium	17.6 mg
Manganese	.1 mg
Phosphorus	134 mg
Potassium	189 mg
Selenium	2.66 mcg
Sodium	189 mg
Zinc	.559 mg
Complex Carbohydrates	3.23 g
Sugars	11.6 g
Mono-Saccharide	.027 g
Di-Saccharide	5.83 g
Alcohol	0 g
Caffeine	0 mg
Water	45.6 g

⊚ Lemon Squares

Calories	33.4
Protein	.719 g
Carbohydrates	4.82 g
Fat—Total	1.21 g
Saturated Fat	.206 g
Monounsaturated Fat	.435 g
Polyunsaturated Fat	.494 g
Omega 3 Fatty Acid	.007 g
Omega 6 Fatty Acid	.489 g
Cholesterol	1.96 mg
Dietary Fiber	.206 g
Total Vitamin A	29.1 RE
A–Retinol	26.7 RE
A–Carotenoid	2.33 RE
Thiamin–B1	.05 mg
Riboflavin–B2	.034 mg
Niacin–B3	.37 mg
Niacin Equivalent	.37 mg
Vitamin B6	.004 mg
Vitamin B12	.006 mcg
Folate	1.91 mcg
Pantothenic	.035 mg
Vitamin C	.178 mg
Vitamin D	.308 mcg
Vitamin E-Alpha E	.204 mg

Calcium	1.7 mg
Copper	.009 mg
Iron	.297 mg
Magnesium	1.49 mg
Manganese	.043 mg
Phosphorus	7.99 mg
Potassium	8.45 mg
Selenium	2.26 mcg
Sodium	10.7 mg
Zinc	.049 mg
Complex Carbohydrates	4.46 g
Sugars	.157 g
Mono-Saccharide	.07 g
Di-Saccharide	.026 g
Alcohol	0 g
Caffeine	0 mg
Water	3.12 g

☺ Maple Bars

Calories	17.3
Protein	.45 g
Carbohydrates	2.66 g
Fat—Total	.512 g
Saturated Fat	.094 g
Monounsaturated Fat	.182 g
Polyunsaturated Fat	.195 g
Omega 3 Fatty Acid	.003 g
Omega 6 Fatty Acid	.192 g
Cholesterol	2.96 mg
Dietary Fiber	.114 g
Total Vitamin A	11.8 RE
A–Retinol	10.9 RE
A–Carotenoid	.859 RE
Thiamin–B1	.028 mg
Riboflavin–B2	.021 mg
Niacin–B3	.206 mg
Niacin Equivalent	.206 mg
Vitamin B6	.003 mg
Vitamin B12	.008 mcg
Folate	1.24 mcg
Pantothenic	.024 mg
Vitamin C	.001 mg
Vitamin D	.121 mcg
Vitamin E-Alpha E	.084 mg

Calcium	1.05 mg
Copper	.005 mg
Iron	.171 mg
Magnesium	.85 mg
Manganese	.024 mg
Phosphorus	5.13 mg
Potassium	4.83 mg
Selenium	1.39 mcg
Sodium	17.8 mg
Zinc	.032 mg
Complex Carbohydrates	2.48 g
Sugars	.072 g
Mono-Saccharide	.04 g
Di-Saccharide	.014 g
Alcohol	0 g
Caffeine	0 mg
Water	1.55 g

⊚ Maple Pudding

Calories	100
Protein	3.98 g
Carbohydrates	6.15 g
Fat—Total	7.12 g
Saturated Fat	1.35 g
Monounsaturated Fat	1.51 g
Polyunsaturated Fat	3.93 g
Omega 3 Fatty Acid	.688 g
Omega 6 Fatty Acid	3.19 g
Cholesterol	1.05 mg
Dietary Fiber	.456 g
Total Vitamin A	7.17 RE
A–Retinol	3.12 RE
A–Carotenoid	4.04 RE
Thiamin–B1	.06 mg
Riboflavin–B2	.118 mg
Niacin–B3	.16 mg
Niacin Equivalent	.16 mg
Vitamin B6	.079 mg
Vitamin B12	.265 mcg
Folate	11.8 mcg
Pantothenic	.325 mg
Vitamin C	.716 mg
Vitamin D	.062 mcg
Vitamin E-Alpha E	.273 mg

Calcium	96.3 mg
Copper	.15 mg
Iron	.301 mg
Magnesium	25.8 mg
Manganese	.317 mg
Phosphorus	104 mg
Potassium	166 mg
Selenium	1.99 mcg
Sodium	41.7 mg
Zinc	.692 mg
Complex Carbohydrates	1.41 g
Sugars	4.28 g
Mono-Saccharide	0 g
Di-Saccharide	.21 g
Alcohol	0 g
Caffeine	.229 mg
Water	40.5 g

⊚ Mock Chocolate Cake

Calories	54.9
Protein	1.24 g
Carbohydrates	6.47 g
Fat—Total	2.66 g
Saturated Fat	.375 g
Monounsaturated Fat	.599 g
Polyunsaturated Fat	1.57 g
Omega 3 Fatty Acid	.013 g
Omega 6 Fatty Acid	1.56 g
Cholesterol	13.4 mg
Dietary Fiber	.651 g
Total Vitamin A	7.87 RE
A–Retinol	7.85 RE
A–Carotenoid	.013 RE
Thiamin–B1	.057 mg
Riboflavin–B2	.059 mg
Niacin–B3	.429 mg
Niacin Equivalent	.429 mg
Vitamin B6	.012 mg
Vitamin B12	.042 mcg
Folate	3.69 mcg
Pantothenic	.078 mg
Vitamin C	.017 mg
Vitamin D	.07 mcg
Vitamin E-Alpha E	1.41 mg

Calcium	21.2 mg
Copper	.017 mg
Iron	.417 mg
Magnesium	2.78 mg
Manganese	.054 mg
Phosphorus	34.8 mg
Potassium	51.6 mg
Selenium	3.44 mcg
Sodium	6.15 mg
Zinc	.106 mg
Complex Carbohydrates	5 g
Sugars	.294 g
Mono-Saccharide	.1 g
Di-Saccharide	.166 g
Alcohol	0 g
Caffeine	0 mg
Water	3.23 g

⊚ Nut Crunch

Calories	35.3
Protein	.594 g
Carbohydrates	1.12 g
Fat—Total	3.32 g
Saturated Fat	.654 g
Monounsaturated Fat	1.48 g
Polyunsaturated Fat	1.02 g
Omega 3 Fatty Acid	.064 g
Omega 6 Fatty Acid	.948 g
Cholesterol	.085 mg
Dietary Fiber	.204 g
Total Vitamin A	21.3 RE
A–Retinol	19.3 RE
A–Carotenoid	1.83 RE
Thiamin–B1	.006 mg
Riboflavin–B2	.014 mg
Niacin–B3	.062 mg
Niacin Equivalent	.062 mg
Vitamin B6	.006 mg
Vitamin B12	.001 mcg
Folate	1.58 mcg
Pantothenic	.012 mg
Vitamin C	.037 mg
Vitamin D	0 mcg
Vitamin E-Alpha E	.554 mg

Calcium	12.6 mg
Copper	.029 mg
Iron	.093 mg
Magnesium	6.55 mg
Manganese	.059 mg
Phosphorus	12 mg
Potassium	17.4 mg
Selenium	.12 mcg
Sodium	.315 mg
Zinc	.089 mg
Complex Carbohydrates	.201 g
Sugars	.499 g
Mono-Saccharide	0 g
Di-Saccharide	.107 g
Alcohol	0 g
Caffeine	0 mg
Water	.487 g

☺ Oatmeal Cookies

Calories	45.8
Protein	.665 g
Carbohydrates	3.29 g
Fat—Total	3.4 g
Saturated Fat	.886 g
Monounsaturated Fat	.63 g
Polyunsaturated Fat	1.77 g
Omega 3 Fatty Acid	.013 g
Omega 6 Fatty Acid	1.76 g
Cholesterol	5.07 mg
Dietary Fiber	.352 g
Total Vitamin A	2.36 RE
A–Retinol	2.27 RE
A–Carotenoid	.089 RE
Thiamin–B1	.031 mg
Riboflavin–B2	.023 mg
Niacin–B3	.189 mg
Niacin Equivalent	.19 mg
Vitamin B6	.007 mg
Vitamin B12	.012 mcg
Folate	1.64 mcg
Pantothenic	.047 mg
Vitamin C	.014 mg
Vitamin D	.015 mcg
Vitamin E-Alpha E	1.59 mg

Calcium	4.54 mg
Copper	.015 mg
Iron	.226 mg
Magnesium	2.96 mg
Manganese	.079 mg
Phosphorus	13.2 mg
Potassium	15.6 mg
Selenium	1.99 mcg
Sodium	18 mg
Zinc	.08 mg
Complex Carbohydrates	2.62 g
Sugars	.322 g
Mono-Saccharide	.042 g
Di-Saccharide	.034 g
Alcohol	0 g
Caffeine	0 mg
Water	6.04 g

✑ Old-Fashioned Candy Canes

Calories	.053
Protein	0 g
Carbohydrates	.014 g
Fat—Total	0 g
Saturated Fat	0 g
Monounsaturated Fat	0 g
Polyunsaturated Fat	0 g
Omega 3 Fatty Acid	0 g
Omega 6 Fatty Acid	0 g
Cholesterol	0 mg
Dietary Fiber	0 g
Total Vitamin A	0 RE
A–Retinol	0 RE
A–Carotenoid	0 RE
Thiamin–B1	0 mg
Riboflavin–B2	0 mg
Niacin–B3	0 mg
Niacin Equivalent	0 mg
Vitamin B6	0 mg
Vitamin B12	0 mcg
Folate	0 mcg
Pantothenic	0 mg
Vitamin C	0 mg
Vitamin D	0 mcg
Vitamin E-Alpha E	0 mg

Calcium	.012 mg
Copper	0 mg
Iron	0 mg
Magnesium	.006 mg
Manganese	0 mg
Phosphorus	0 mg
Potassium	.653 mg
Selenium	0 mcg
Sodium	.076 mg
Zinc	0 mg
Complex Carbohydrates	0 g
Sugars	.014 g
Mono-Saccharide	0 g
Di-Saccharide	0 g
Alcohol	0 g
Caffeine	0 mg
Water	.615 g

⊚ Orange Pound Cake

Calories	82.9
Protein	2.67 g
Carbohydrates	9.61 g
Fat—Total	3.68 g
Saturated Fat	.767 g
Monounsaturated Fat	1.35 g
Polyunsaturated Fat	1.23 g
Omega 3 Fatty Acid	.023 g
Omega 6 Fatty Acid	1.21 g
Cholesterol	47.3 mg
Dietary Fiber	.398 g
Total Vitamin A	83.9 RE
A–Retinol	78.6 RE
A–Carotenoid	5.16 RE
Thiamin–B1	.103 mg
Riboflavin–B2	.118 mg
Niacin–B3	.727 mg
Niacin Equivalent	.727 mg
Vitamin B6	.021 mg
Vitamin B12	.115 mcg
Folate	8.43 mcg
Pantothenic	.196 mg
Vitamin C	.006 mg
Vitamin D	.861 mcg
Vitamin E-Alpha E	.536 mg

Calcium	23.9 mg
Copper	.019 mg
Iron	.754 mg
Magnesium	3.99 mg
Manganese	.087 mg
Phosphorus	58.4 mg
Potassium	64.2 mg
Selenium	7.54 mcg
Sodium	36.8 mg
Zinc	.211 mg
Complex Carbohydrates	8.83 g
Sugars	.37 g
Mono-Saccharide	.247 g
Di-Saccharide	.040 g
Alcohol	0 g
Caffeine	0 mg
Water	13.5 g

⊘ Orange Sticks

Calories	24.3
Protein	.44 g
Carbohydrates	2.04 g
Fat—Total	1.76 g
Saturated Fat	.442 g
Monounsaturated Fat	.546 g
Polyunsaturated Fat	.683 g
Omega 3 Fatty Acid	.077 g
Omega 6 Fatty Acid	.602 g
Cholesterol	.048 mg
Dietary Fiber	.219 g
Total Vitamin A	12.6 RE
A–Retinol	9.17 RE
A–Carotenoid	1.23 RE
Thiamin–B1	.012 mg
Riboflavin–B2	.012 mg
Niacin–B3	.04 mg
Niacin Equivalent	.033 mg
Vitamin B6	.012 mg
Vitamin B12	.012 mcg
Folate	1.48 mcg
Pantothenic	.04 mg
Vitamin C	.655 mg
Vitamin D	0 mcg
Vitamin E-Alpha E	.177 mg

Calcium	11 mg
Copper	.028 mg
Iron	.121 mg
Magnesium	4.39 mg
Manganese	.064 mg
Phosphorus	17.3 mg
Potassium	37.5 mg
Selenium	.422 mcg
Sodium	4.37 mg
Zinc	.073 mg
Complex Carbohydrates	.325 g
Sugars	1.16 g
Mono-Saccharide	.926 g
Di-Saccharide	.073 g
Alcohol	0 g
Caffeine	.632 mg
Water	1.79 g

⊚ Peach Pie

Calories	52
Protein	.935 g
Carbohydrates	12.2 g
Fat—Total	.425 g
Saturated Fat	.287 g
Monounsaturated Fat	.052 g
Polyunsaturated Fat	.058 g
Omega 3 Fatty Acid	.005 g
Omega 6 Fatty Acid	.054 g
Cholesterol	0 mg
Dietary Fiber	1.63 g
Total Vitamin A	46.6 RE
A–Retinol	0 RE
A–Carotenoid	46.6 RE
Thiamin–B1	.039 mg
Riboflavin–B2	.051 mg
Niacin–B3	1.03 mg
Niacin Equivalent	1.02 mg
Vitamin B6	.017 mg
Vitamin B12	0 mcg
Folate	3.77 mcg
Pantothenic	.159 mg
Vitamin C	5.83 mg
Vitamin D	0 mcg
Vitamin E-Alpha E	.609 mg

Calcium	4.83 mg
Copper	.063 mg
Iron	.24 mg
Magnesium	6.69 mg
Manganese	.062 mg
Phosphorus	13.7 mg
Potassium	172 mg
Selenium	2.17 mcg
Sodium	.384 mg
Zinc	.142 mg
Complex Carbohydrates	2.23 g
Sugars	7.88 g
Mono-Saccharide	2.08 g
Di-Saccharide	5.36 g
Alcohol	0 g
Caffeine	.632 mg
Water	76 g

◎ Peach Tarts

Calories	54.4
Protein	.819 g
Carbohydrates	9.45 g
Fat—Total	1.56 g
Saturated Fat	.256 g
Monounsaturated Fat	.562 g
Polyunsaturated Fat	.655 g
Omega 3 Fatty Acid	.01 g
Omega 6 Fatty Acid	.647 g
Cholesterol	0 mg
Dietary Fiber	.574 g
Total Vitamin A	47.9 RE
A–Retinol	34.4 RE
A–Carotenoid	13.3 RE
Thiamin–B1	.053 mg
Riboflavin–B2	.041 mg
Niacin–B3	.563 mg
Niacin Equivalent	.563 mg
Vitamin B6	.011 mg
Vitamin B12	.002 mcg
Folate	2.34 mcg
Pantothenic	.07 mg
Vitamin C	1.34 mg
Vitamin D	.403 mcg
Vitamin E-Alpha E	.393 mg

Calcium	3.3 mg
Copper	.024 mg
Iron	.349 mg
Magnesium	3.41 mg
Manganese	.06 mg
Phosphorus	10.6 mg
Potassium	61.1 mg
Selenium	2.39 mcg
Sodium	14.4 mg
Zinc	.076 mg
Complex Carbohydrates	5.54 g
Sugars	3.18 g
Mono-Saccharide	.516 g
Di-Saccharide	1.23 g
Alcohol	0 g
Caffeine	0 mg
Water	21.8 g

⑨ Peach Upside-Down Cake

Calories	23.9
Protein	.752 g
Carbohydrates	4.16 g
Fat—Total	.476 g
Saturated Fat	.06 g
Monounsaturated Fat	.096 g
Polyunsaturated Fat	.302 g
Omega 3 Fatty Acid	.003 g
Omega 6 Fatty Acid	.295 g
Cholesterol	.069 mg
Dietary Fiber	.259 g
Total Vitamin A	4.18 RE
A–Retinol	1.2 RE
A–Carotenoid	2.98 RE
Thiamin–B1	.037 mg
Riboflavin–B2	.036 mg
Niacin–B3	.316 mg
Niacin Equivalent	.313 mg
Vitamin B6	.006 mg
Vitamin B12	.023 mcg
Folate	1.34 mcg
Pantothenic	.054 mg
Vitamin C	.785 mg
Vitamin D	.02 mcg
Vitamin E-Alpha E	.297 mg

Calcium	7.29 mg
Copper	.011 mg
Iron	.29 mg
Magnesium	1.93 mg
Manganese	.031 mg
Phosphorus	9.3 mg
Potassium	27.6 mg
Selenium	.729 mcg
Sodium	5.98 mg
Zinc	.061 mg
Complex Carbohydrates	2.8 g
Sugars	1.05 g
Mono-Saccharide	.149 g
Di-Saccharide	.427 g
Alcohol	0 g
Caffeine	0 mg
Water	12.9 g

⊚ Peanut Butter Balls

Calories	16.4
Protein	.451 g
Carbohydrates	.649 g
Fat—Total	1.47 g
Saturated Fat	.705 g
Monounsaturated Fat	.424 g
Polyunsaturated Fat	.258 g
Omega 3 Fatty Acid	0 g
Omega 6 Fatty Acid	.258 g
Cholesterol	0 mg
Dietary Fiber	.294 g
Total Vitamin A	0 RE
A–Retinol	0 RE
A–Carotenoid	0 RE
Thiamin–B1	.008 mg
Riboflavin–B2	.002 mg
Niacin–B3	.227 mg
Niacin Equivalent	.227 mg
Vitamin B6	.007 mg
Vitamin B12	0 mcg
Folate	2.85 mcg
Pantothenic	.028 mg
Vitamin C	.066 mg
Vitamin D	0 mcg
Vitamin E-Alpha E	.135 mg

Calcium	1.15 mg
Copper	.019 mg
Iron	.085 mg
Magnesium	3.46 mg
Manganese	.063 mg
Phosphorus	8.01 mg
Potassium	17.7 mg
Selenium	.513 mcg
Sodium	.496 mg
Zinc	.075 mg
Complex Carbohydrates	.118 g
Sugars	.244 g
Mono-Saccharide	.068 g
Di-Saccharide	.002 g
Alcohol	0 g
Caffeine	0 mg
Water	.964 g

⑨ Peanut Butter and Banana Fudge

Calories	14.2
Protein	.545 g
Carbohydrates	1.15 g
Fat—Total	.942 g
Saturated Fat	.174 g
Monounsaturated Fat	.42 g
Polyunsaturated Fat	.258 g
Omega 3 Fatty Acid	.002 g
Omega 6 Fatty Acid	.256 g
Cholesterol	0 mg
Dietary Fiber	.18 g
Total Vitamin A	.094 RE
A–Retinol	0 RE
A–Carotenoid	.094 RE
Thiamin–B1	.006 mg
Riboflavin–B2	.004 mg
Niacin–B3	.297 mg
Niacin Equivalent	.297 mg
Vitamin B6	.023 mg
Vitamin B12	0 mcg
Folate	1.88 mcg
Pantothenic	.034 mg
Vitamin C	.325 mg
Vitamin D	0 mcg
Vitamin E-Alpha E	.005 mg

Calcium	.929 mg
Copper	.018 mg
Iron	.047 mg
Magnesium	4.13 mg
Manganese	.034 mg
Phosphorus	7.64 mg
Potassium	26.7 mg
Selenium	.035 mcg
Sodium	.462 mg
Zinc	.063 mg
Complex Carbohydrates	.652 g
Sugars	.385 g
Mono-Saccharide	.11 g
Di-Saccharide	.239 g
Alcohol	0 g
Caffeine	0 mg
Water	3.18 g

❂ Peanut Butter Bars

Calories	77.5
Protein	2.56 g
Carbohydrates	6.7 g
Fat—Total	4.75 g
Saturated Fat	.769 g
Monounsaturated Fat	2.25 g
Polyunsaturated Fat	1.45 g
Omega 3 Fatty Acid	.009 g
Omega 6 Fatty Acid	1.44 g
Cholesterol	11.8 mg
Dietary Fiber	.663 g
Total Vitamin A	21 RE
A–Retinol	19.6 RE
A–Carotenoid	1.29 RE
Thiamin–B1	.084 mg
Riboflavin–B2	.055 mg
Niacin–B3	1.26 mg
Niacin Equivalent	1.26 mg
Vitamin B6	.023 mg
Vitamin B12	.029 mcg
Folate	12.3 mcg
Pantothenic	.154 mg
Vitamin C	.001 mg
Vitamin D	.036 mcg
Vitamin E-Alpha E	.719 mg

Calcium	6.08 mg
Copper	.053 mg
Iron	.505 mg
Magnesium	12.9 mg
Manganese	.179 mg
Phosphorus	35.2 mg
Potassium	52.7 mg
Selenium	3.68 mcg
Sodium	4.05 mg
Zinc	.288 mg
Complex Carbohydrates	5.58 g
Sugars	.45 g
Mono-Saccharide	.11 g
Di-Saccharide	.28 g
Alcohol	0 g
Caffeine	0 mg
Water	3.31 g

☺ Peanut Butter Cookies

Calories	53.1
Protein	2.26 g
Carbohydrates	1.97 g
Fat—Total	4.43 g
Saturated Fat	.673 g
Monounsaturated Fat	2.16 g
Polyunsaturated Fat	1.36 g
Omega 3 Fatty Acid	.001 g
Omega 6 Fatty Acid	1.36 g
Cholesterol	6.25 mg
Dietary Fiber	.563 g
Total Vitamin A	2.81 RE
A–Retinol	2.8 RE
A–Carotenoid	0 RE
Thiamin–B1	.038 mg
Riboflavin–B2	.017 mg
Niacin–B3	1.15 mg
Niacin Equivalent	1.15 mg
Vitamin B6	.036 mg
Vitamin B12	.015 mcg
Folate	13.1 mcg
Pantothenic	.138 mg
Vitamin C	0 mg
Vitamin D	.019 mcg
Vitamin E-Alpha E	.653 mg

Calcium	6.69 mg
Copper	.058 mg
Iron	.216 mg
Magnesium	15.2 mg
Manganese	.178 mg
Phosphorus	33.3 mg
Potassium	58 mg
Selenium	1.09 mcg
Sodium	2.36 mg
Zinc	.299 mg
Complex Carbohydrates	.632 g
Sugars	.732 g
Mono-Saccharide	.018 g
Di-Saccharide	0 g
Alcohol	0 g
Caffeine	0 mg
Water	1.23 g

⊚ **Peanut Butter and Cream Cheese Kisses**

Calories	36
Protein	1.79 g
Carbohydrates	2.4 g
Fat—Total	2.21 g
Saturated Fat	.854 g
Monounsaturated Fat	.755 g
Polyunsaturated Fat	.461 g
Omega 3 Fatty Acid	.002 g
Omega 6 Fatty Acid	.458 g
Cholesterol	.975 mg
Dietary Fiber	.212 g
Total Vitamin A	12.1 RE
A–Retinol	0 RE
A–Carotenoid	0 RE
Thiamin–B1	.004 mg
Riboflavin–B2	.012 mg
Niacin–B3	.438 mg
Niacin Equivalent	.438 mg
Vitamin B6	.014 mg
Vitamin B12	0 mcg
Folate	2.94 mcg
Pantothenic	.031 mg
Vitamin C	0 mg
Vitamin D	0 mcg
Vitamin E-Alpha E	.24 mg

Calcium	19.3 mg
Copper	.017 mg
Iron	.087 mg
Magnesium	5.09 mg
Manganese	.059 mg
Phosphorus	10.1 mg
Potassium	23.9 mg
Selenium	.24 mcg
Sodium	26 mg
Zinc	.089 mg
Complex Carbohydrates	.221 g
Sugars	1.23 g
Mono-Saccharide	.038 g
Di-Saccharide	.212 g
Alcohol	0 g
Caffeine	0 mg
Water	.036 g

◉ Peanut Butter Cups

Calories	91.9
Protein	3.42 g
Carbohydrates	7.25 g
Fat—Total	5.85 g
Saturated Fat	2.81 g
Monounsaturated Fat	1.51 g
Polyunsaturated Fat	.922 g
Omega 3 Fatty Acid	.005 g
Omega 6 Fatty Acid	.916 g
Cholesterol	.907 mg
Dietary Fiber	.422 g
Total Vitamin A	.73 RE
A–Retinol	0 RE
A–Carotenoid	0 RE
Thiamin–B1	.01 mg
Riboflavin–B2	.006 mg
Niacin–B3	.908 mg
Niacin Equivalent	.908 mg
Vitamin B6	.028 mg
Vitamin B12	0 mcg
Folate	5 mcg
Pantothenic	.059 mg
Vitamin C	0 mg
Vitamin D	0 mcg
Vitamin E-Alpha E	0 mg

Calcium	74 mg
Copper	.042 mg
Iron	.224 mg
Magnesium	11.5 mg
Manganese	.102 mg
Phosphorus	22.4 mg
Potassium	44.4 mg
Selenium	0 mcg
Sodium	1.09 mg
Zinc	.192 mg
Complex Carbohydrates	.398 g
Sugars	4.4 g
Mono-Saccharide	.077 g
Di-Saccharide	.422 g
Alcohol	0 g
Caffeine	0 mg
Water	.077 g

☯ Peanut Butter Fudge

Calories	10.9
Protein	.414 g
Carbohydrates	.698 g
Fat—Total	.797 g
Saturated Fat	.11 g
Monounsaturated Fat	.395 g
Polyunsaturated Fat	.252 g
Omega 3 Fatty Acid	0 g
Omega 6 Fatty Acid	.252 g
Cholesterol	0 mg
Dietary Fiber	.129 g
Total Vitamin A	0 RE
A–Retinol	0 RE
A–Carotenoid	0 RE
Thiamin–B1	.009 mg
Riboflavin–B2	.002 mg
Niacin–B3	.239 mg
Niacin Equivalent	.239 mg
Vitamin B6	.011 mg
Vitamin B12	0 mcg
Folate	2.48 mcg
Pantothenic	.031 mg
Vitamin C	.131 mg
Vitamin D	0 mcg
Vitamin E-Alpha E	.121 mg

Calcium	1.01 mg
Copper	.014 mg
Iron	.042 mg
Magnesium	3.17 mg
Manganese	.036 mg
Phosphorus	6.46 mg
Potassium	16.4 mg
Selenium	.133 mcg
Sodium	.185 mg
Zinc	.058 mg
Complex Carbohydrates	.423 g
Sugars	.138 g
Mono-Saccharide	0 g
Di-Saccharide	0 g
Alcohol	0 g
Caffeine	0 mg
Water	1.4 g

⑨ Peanut Butter-Potato Pinwheels

Calories	21.7
Protein	.85 g
Carbohydrates	1.1 g
Fat—Total	1.7 g
Saturated Fat	.327 g
Monounsaturated Fat	.805 g
Polyunsaturated Fat	.493 g
Omega 3 Fatty Acid	.003 g
Omega 6 Fatty Acid	.489 g
Cholesterol	0 mg
Dietary Fiber	.25 g
Total Vitamin A	0 RE
A–Retinol	0 RE
A–Carotenoid	0 RE
Thiamin–B1	.006 mg
Riboflavin–B2	.004 mg
Niacin–B3	.491 mg
Niacin Equivalent	.491 mg
Vitamin B6	.02 mg
Vitamin B12	0 mcg
Folate	3.3 mcg
Pantothenic	.042 mg
Vitamin C	.133 mg
Vitamin D	0 mcg
Vitamin E-Alpha E	.257 mg

Calcium	1.55 mg
Copper	.021 mg
Iron	.07 mg
Magnesium	5.79 mg
Manganese	.066 mg
Phosphorus	11.5 mg
Potassium	33.1 mg
Selenium	.27 mcg
Sodium	.671 mg
Zinc	.1 mg
Complex Carbohydrates	.545 g
Sugars	.295 g
Mono-Saccharide	.041 g
Di-Saccharide	.226 g
Alcohol	0 g
Caffeine	0 mg
Water	1.45 g

◉ Pie Crust

Calories	68.2
Protein	1.29 g
Carbohydrates	9.54 g
Fat—Total	2.69 g
Saturated Fat	.661 g
Monounsaturated Fat	1.15 g
Polyunsaturated Fat	.72 g
Omega 3 Fatty Acid	.044 g
Omega 6 Fatty Acid	.676 g
Cholesterol	0 mg
Dietary Fiber	.409 g
Total Vitamin A	0 RE
A–Retinol	0 RE
A–Carotenoid	0 RE
Thiamin–B1	.098 mg
Riboflavin–B2	.062 mg
Niacin–B3	.738 mg
Niacin Equivalent	.738 mg
Vitamin B6	.006 mg
Vitamin B12	0 mcg
Folate	3.25 mcg
Pantothenic	.055 mg
Vitamin C	0 mg
Vitamin D	0 mcg
Vitamin E-Alpha E	.423 mg

Calcium	1.88 mg
Copper	.018 mg
Iron	.581 mg
Magnesium	2.75 mg
Manganese	.086 mg
Phosphorus	13.5 mg
Potassium	13.4 mg
Selenium	4.24 mcg
Sodium	.25 mg
Zinc	.088 mg
Complex Carbohydrates	8.91 g
Sugars	.213 g
Mono-Saccharide	.113 g
Di-Saccharide	.05 g
Alcohol	0 g
Caffeine	0 mg
Water	1.49 g

❂ Pineapple Pie

Calories	92.8
Protein	1.69 g
Carbohydrates	12.4 g
Fat—Total	4.21 g
Saturated Fat	2.13 g
Monounsaturated Fat	1.46 g
Polyunsaturated Fat	.317 g
Omega 3 Fatty Acid	.059 g
Omega 6 Fatty Acid	.255 g
Cholesterol	9.44 mg
Dietary Fiber	.512 g
Total Vitamin A	28.7 RE
A–Retinol	25.4 RE
A–Carotenoid	3.29 RE
Thiamin–B1	.05 mg
Riboflavin–B2	.083 mg
Niacin–B3	.578 mg
Niacin Equivalent	.578 mg
Vitamin B6	.026 mg
Vitamin B12	.081 mcg
Folate	6.4 mcg
Pantothenic	.176 mg
Vitamin C	2.62 mg
Vitamin D	.064 mcg
Vitamin E-Alpha E	.168 mg

Calcium	32.2 mg
Copper	.047 mg
Iron	.533 mg
Magnesium	8.81 mg
Manganese	.366 mg
Phosphorus	40.9 mg
Potassium	71.5 mg
Selenium	1.62 mcg
Sodium	87.7 mg
Zinc	.242 mg
Complex Carbohydrates	3.38 g
Sugars	8.55 g
Mono-Saccharide	.775 g
Di-Saccharide	1.51 g
Alcohol	0 g
Caffeine	.137 mg
Water	35.4 g

⊚ **Potato Bon Bons**

Calories	27.3
Protein	.748 g
Carbohydrates	4.24 g
Fat—Total	.842 g
Saturated Fat	.734 g
Monounsaturated Fat	0 g
Polyunsaturated Fat	.005 g
Omega 3 Fatty Acid	.001 g
Omega 6 Fatty Acid	.004 g
Cholesterol	.302 mg
Dietary Fiber	.141 g
Total Vitamin A	.243 RE
A–Retinol	0 RE
A–Carotenoid	0 RE
Thiamin–B1	.011 mg
Riboflavin–B2	.002 mg
Niacin–B3	.142 mg
Niacin Equivalent	.142 mg
Vitamin B6	.029 mg
Vitamin B12	0 mcg
Folate	.96 mcg
Pantothenic	.055 mg
Vitamin C	.799 mg
Vitamin D	0 mcg
Vitamin E-Alpha E	.005 mg

Calcium	24.8 mg
Copper	.018 mg
Iron	.068 mg
Magnesium	2.16 mg
Manganese	.015 mg
Phosphorus	4.32 mg
Potassium	35.4 mg
Selenium	.086 mcg
Sodium	.541 mg
Zinc	.029 mg
Complex Carbohydrates	1.86 g
Sugars	1.41 g
Mono-Saccharide	0 g
Di-Saccharide	0 g
Alcohol	0 g
Caffeine	0 mg
Water	8.4 g

◎ Pralines

Calories	39.2
Protein	.531 g
Carbohydrates	1.13 g
Fat—Total	3.89 g
Saturated Fat	.368 g
Monounsaturated Fat	2.36 g
Polyunsaturated Fat	.976 g
Omega 3 Fatty Acid	.037 g
Omega 6 Fatty Acid	.939 g
Cholesterol	.134 mg
Dietary Fiber	.24 g
Total Vitamin A	5.37 RE
A–Retinol	4.3 RE
A–Carotenoid	1.06 RE
Thiamin–B1	.045 mg
Riboflavin–B2	.013 mg
Niacin–B3	.048 mg
Niacin Equivalent	.048 mg
Vitamin B6	.011 mg
Vitamin B12	.009 mcg
Folate	2.22 mcg
Pantothenic	.099 mg
Vitamin C	.142 mg
Vitamin D	.002 mcg
Vitamin E-Alpha E	.22 mg

Calcium	6.38 mg
Copper	.061 mg
Iron	.113 mg
Magnesium	7.04 mg
Manganese	.234 mg
Phosphorus	18.5 mg
Potassium	26.2 mg
Selenium	.346 mcg
Sodium	23.7 mg
Zinc	.3 mg
Complex Carbohydrates	.479 g
Sugars	.409 g
Mono-Saccharide	.008 g
Di-Saccharide	.349 g
Alcohol	0 g
Caffeine	0 mg
Water	3.78 g

☺ Pretzels

Calories	71.6
Protein	2.25 g
Carbohydrates	8.3 g
Fat—Total	3.33 g
Saturated Fat	2.92 g
Monounsaturated Fat	0 g
Polyunsaturated Fat	0 g
Omega 3 Fatty Acid	0 g
Omega 6 Fatty Acid	0 g
Cholesterol	1.21 mg
Dietary Fiber	0 g
Total Vitamin A	.973 RE
A–Retinol	0 RE
A–Carotenoid	0 RE
Thiamin–B1	0 mg
Riboflavin–B2	0 mg
Niacin–B3	0 mg
Niacin Equivalent	0 mg
Vitamin B6	0 mg
Vitamin B12	0 mcg
Folate	0 mcg
Pantothenic	0 mg
Vitamin C	0 mg
Vitamin D	0 mcg
Vitamin E-Alpha E	0 mg

Calcium	95.7 mg
Copper	0 mg
Iron	.137 mg
Magnesium	0 mg
Manganese	0 mg
Phosphorus	0 mg
Potassium	0 mg
Selenium	0 mcg
Sodium	0 mg
Zinc	0 mg
Complex Carbohydrates	0 g
Sugars	5.2 g
Mono-Saccharide	0 g
Di-Saccharide	0 g
Alcohol	0 g
Caffeine	0 mg
Water	0 g

☻ Prune Purée

Calories	454
Protein	4.45 g
Carbohydrates	119 g
Fat—Total	.885 g
Saturated Fat	.069 g
Monounsaturated Fat	.579 g
Polyunsaturated Fat	.19 g
Omega 3 Fatty Acid	0 g
Omega 6 Fatty Acid	.19 g
Cholesterol	0 mg
Dietary Fiber	15.7 g
Total Vitamin A	338 RE
A–Retinol	0 RE
A–Carotenoid	338 RE
Thiamin–B1	.141 mg
Riboflavin–B2	.278 mg
Niacin–B3	3.35 mg
Niacin Equivalent	3.35 mg
Vitamin B6	.45 mg
Vitamin B12	0 mcg
Folate	6.3 mcg
Pantothenic	.789 mg
Vitamin C	5.61 mg
Vitamin D	0 mcg
Vitamin E-Alpha E	2.27 mg

Calcium	87 mg
Copper	.732 mg
Iron	4.24 mg
Magnesium	76.5 mg
Manganese	.4 mg
Phosphorus	147 mg
Potassium	1269 mg
Selenium	4.45 mcg
Sodium	63.5 mg
Zinc	.907 mg
Complex Carbohydrates	0 g
Sugars	73.1 g
Mono-Saccharide	63.2 g
Di-Saccharide	1.36 g
Alcohol	0 g
Caffeine	0 mg
Water	70.7 g

☺ Pumpkin Pie

Calories	58.1
Protein	3.29 g
Carbohydrates	7.03 g
Fat—Total	2.11 g
Saturated Fat	.916 g
Monounsaturated Fat	.64 g
Polyunsaturated Fat	.225 g
Omega 3 Fatty Acid	.019 g
Omega 6 Fatty Acid	.207 g
Cholesterol	64.8 mg
Dietary Fiber	1.27 g
Total Vitamin A	1061 RE
A–Retinol	58.9 RE
A–Carotenoid	1002 RE
Thiamin–B1	.031 mg
Riboflavin–B2	.135 mg
Niacin–B3	.211 mg
Niacin Equivalent	.212 mg
Vitamin B6	.059 mg
Vitamin B12	.216 mcg
Folate	15 mcg
Pantothenic	.559 mg
Vitamin C	2.23 mg
Vitamin D	.694 mcg
Vitamin E-Alpha E	.629 mg

Calcium	92.7 mg
Copper	.054 mg
Iron	.882 mg
Magnesium	17.8 mg
Manganese	.073 mg
Phosphorus	90 mg
Potassium	183 mg
Selenium	3.45 mcg
Sodium	34.1 mg
Zinc	.463 mg
Complex Carbohydrates	.904 g
Sugars	4.86 g
Mono-Saccharide	.089 g
Di-Saccharide	2.91 g
Alcohol	0 g
Caffeine	0 mg
Water	64.3 g

☺ **Pumpkin Squares**

Calories	1.57
Protein	.172 g
Carbohydrates	.191 g
Fat—Total	.003 g
Saturated Fat	.001 g
Monounsaturated Fat	0 g
Polyunsaturated Fat	0 g
Omega 3 Fatty Acid	0 g
Omega 6 Fatty Acid	0 g
Cholesterol	.187 mg
Dietary Fiber	.028 g
Total Vitamin A	36.1 RE
A–Retinol	0 RE
A–Carotenoid	33.1 RE
Thiamin–B1	.001 mg
Riboflavin–B2	.005 mg
Niacin–B3	.013 mg
Niacin Equivalent	.013 mg
Vitamin B6	.001 mg
Vitamin B12	0 mcg
Folate	.26 mcg
Pantothenic	.006 mg
Vitamin C	.145 mg
Vitamin D	0 mcg
Vitamin E-Alpha E	.022 mg

Calcium	.504 mg
Copper	.003 mg
Iron	.019 mg
Magnesium	.284 mg
Manganese	.004 mg
Phosphorus	.926 mg
Potassium	7.09 mg
Selenium	.031 mcg
Sodium	6.4 mg
Zinc	.007 mg
Complex Carbohydrates	.002 g
Sugars	.1 g
Mono-Saccharide	.068 g
Di-Saccharide	.03 g
Alcohol	0 g
Caffeine	0 mg
Water	2.87 g

☺ Pumpkin Tarts

Calories	12.3
Protein	.75 g
Carbohydrates	.973 g
Fat—Total	.63 g
Saturated Fat	.35 g
Monounsaturated Fat	.167 g
Polyunsaturated Fat	.046 g
Omega 3 Fatty Acid	.007 g
Omega 6 Fatty Acid	.039 g
Cholesterol	11.5 mg
Dietary Fiber	.172 g
Total Vitamin A	143 RE
A–Retinol	6.42 RE
A–Carotenoid	136 RE
Thiamin–B1	.005 mg
Riboflavin–B2	.033 mg
Niacin–B3	.031 mg
Niacin Equivalent	.031 mg
Vitamin B6	.01 mg
Vitamin B12	.05 mcg
Folate	2.28 mcg
Pantothenic	.077 mg
Vitamin C	.316 mg
Vitamin D	.094 mcg
Vitamin E-Alpha E	.093 mg

Calcium	10.2 mg
Copper	.008 mg
Iron	.126 mg
Magnesium	2.66 mg
Manganese	.01 mg
Phosphorus	12.6 mg
Potassium	27.2 mg
Selenium	1.24 mcg
Sodium	9.11 mg
Zinc	.062 mg
Complex Carbohydrates	.122 g
Sugars	.679 g
Mono-Saccharide	.047 g
Di-Saccharide	.285 g
Alcohol	0 g
Caffeine	0 mg
Water	14.4 g

⊚ Raisin Clusters

Calories	35.9
Protein	1 g
Carbohydrates	5.05 g
Fat—Total	1.4 g
Saturated Fat	1.22 g
Monounsaturated Fat	0 g
Polyunsaturated Fat	.003 g
Omega 3 Fatty Acid	.001 g
Omega 6 Fatty Acid	.002 g
Cholesterol	.504 mg
Dietary Fiber	.07 g
Total Vitamin A	.421 RE
A–Retinol	0 RE
A–Carotenoid	.016 RE
Thiamin–B1	.003 mg
Riboflavin–B2	.002 mg
Niacin–B3	.017 mg
Niacin Equivalent	.017 mg
Vitamin B6	.005 mg
Vitamin B12	0 mcg
Folate	.067 mcg
Pantothenic	.001 mg
Vitamin C	.067 mg
Vitamin D	0 mcg
Vitamin E-Alpha E	.014 mg

Calcium	40.8 mg
Copper	.006 mg
Iron	.099 mg
Magnesium	.665 mg
Manganese	.006 mg
Phosphorus	1.96 mg
Potassium	15.1 mg
Selenium	.134 mcg
Sodium	.242 mg
Zinc	.005 mg
Complex Carbohydrates	0 g
Sugars	3.68 g
Mono-Saccharide	1.31 g
Di-Saccharide	0 g
Alcohol	0 g
Caffeine	0 mg
Water	.31 g

⑨ Rascal Raspberries

Calories	49.2
Protein	1.52 g
Carbohydrates	5.85 g
Fat—Total	2.23 g
Saturated Fat	1.95 g
Monounsaturated Fat	.001 g
Polyunsaturated Fat	.009 g
Omega 3 Fatty Acid	.003 g
Omega 6 Fatty Acid	.006 g
Cholesterol	.806 mg
Dietary Fiber	.108 g
Total Vitamin A	1 RE
A–Retinol	0 RE
A–Carotenoid	.356 RE
Thiamin–B1	.001 mg
Riboflavin–B2	.002 mg
Niacin–B3	.025 mg
Niacin Equivalent	0 mg
Vitamin B6	.002 mg
Vitamin B12	0 mcg
Folate	.711 mcg
Pantothenic	.007 mg
Vitamin C	.684 mg
Vitamin D	0 mcg
Vitamin E-Alpha E	.012 mg

Calcium	64.4 mg
Copper	.002 mg
Iron	.107 mg
Magnesium	.491 mg
Manganese	.028 mg
Phosphorus	.329 mg
Potassium	4.16 mg
Selenium	.014 mcg
Sodium	.001 mg
Zinc	.013 mg
Complex Carbohydrates	0 g
Sugars	3.73 g
Mono-Saccharide	.183 g
Di-Saccharide	.076 g
Alcohol	0 g
Caffeine	0 mg
Water	2.4 g

⊚ Raspberry Crunch

Calories	55.9
Protein	1.06 g
Carbohydrates	5.24 g
Fat—Total	3.45 g
Saturated Fat	.484 g
Monounsaturated Fat	1.61 g
Polyunsaturated Fat	1.16 g
Omega 3 Fatty Acid	.027 g
Omega 6 Fatty Acid	1.13 g
Cholesterol	8.88 mg
Dietary Fiber	.339 g
Total Vitamin A	51.4 RE
A–Retinol	47 RE
A–Carotenoid	4.29 RE
Thiamin–B1	.066 mg
Riboflavin–B2	.045 mg
Niacin–B3	.385 mg
Niacin Equivalent	.374 mg
Vitamin B6	.01 mg
Vitamin B12	.023 mcg
Folate	3.68 mcg
Pantothenic	.092 mg
Vitamin C	.365 mg
Vitamin D	.53 mcg
Vitamin E-Alpha E	.401 mg

Calcium	3.86 mg
Copper	.033 mg
Iron	.359 mg
Magnesium	4.42 mg
Manganese	.143 mg
Phosphorus	16.7 mg
Potassium	25 mg
Selenium	2.78 mcg
Sodium	20 mg
Zinc	.181 mg
Complex Carbohydrates	4.45 g
Sugars	.467 g
Mono-Saccharide	.166 g
Di-Saccharide	.139 g
Alcohol	0 g
Caffeine	0 mg
Water	11.2 g

⊚ Spice Delight

Calories	38.5
Protein	.728 g
Carbohydrates	4.84 g
Fat—Total	1.77 g
Saturated Fat	.305 g
Monounsaturated Fat	.643 g
Polyunsaturated Fat	.726 g
Omega 3 Fatty Acid	.01 g
Omega 6 Fatty Acid	.718 g
Cholesterol	1.96 mg
Dietary Fiber	.23 g
Total Vitamin A	43.2 RE
A–Retinol	39.6 RE
A–Carotenoid	3.5 RE
Thiamin–B1	.05 mg
Riboflavin–B2	.034 mg
Niacin–B3	.371 mg
Niacin Equivalent	.371 mg
Vitamin B6	.004 mg
Vitamin B12	.007 mcg
Folate	1.87 mcg
Pantothenic	.035 mg
Vitamin C	.018 mg
Vitamin D	.459 mcg
Vitamin E-Alpha E	.291 mg

Calcium	2.38 mg
Copper	.01 mg
Iron	.311 mg
Magnesium	1.6 mg
Manganese	.053 mg
Phosphorus	8.26 mg
Potassium	8.81 mg
Selenium	2.27 mcg
Sodium	15.7 mg
Zinc	.051 mg
Complex Carbohydrates	4.47 g
Sugars	.143 g
Mono-Saccharide	.062 g
Di-Saccharide	.025 g
Alcohol	0 g
Caffeine	0 mg
Water	3.61 g

⊚ Striped Candy Canes

Calories	5.08
Protein	1.06 g
Carbohydrates	.105 g
Fat—Total	0 g
Saturated Fat	0 g
Monounsaturated Fat	0 g
Polyunsaturated Fat	0 g
Omega 3 Fatty Acid	0 g
Omega 6 Fatty Acid	0 g
Cholesterol	0 mg
Dietary Fiber	0 g
Total Vitamin A	0 RE
A–Retinol	0 RE
A–Carotenoid	0 RE
Thiamin–B1	.001 mg
Riboflavin–B2	.046 mg
Niacin–B3	.009 mg
Niacin Equivalent	.009 mg
Vitamin B6	0 mg
Vitamin B12	.02 mcg
Folate	.304 mcg
Pantothenic	.012 mg
Vitamin C	0 mg
Vitamin D	0 mcg
Vitamin E-Alpha E	0 mg

Calcium	.608 mg
Copper	.001 mg
Iron	.003 mg
Magnesium	1.11 mg
Manganese	0 mg
Phosphorus	1.32 mg
Potassium	14.5 mg
Selenium	1.78 mcg
Sodium	16.6 mg
Zinc	.001 mg
Complex Carbohydrates	0 g
Sugars	.105 g
Mono-Saccharide	.105 g
Di-Saccharide	0 g
Alcohol	0 g
Caffeine	0 mg
Water	8.89 g

⑨ Stuffed Dates

Calories	42
Protein	.603 g
Carbohydrates	7.46 g
Fat—Total	1.54 g
Saturated Fat	.177 g
Monounsaturated Fat	.865 g
Polyunsaturated Fat	.419 g
Omega 3 Fatty Acid	.008 g
Omega 6 Fatty Acid	.407 g
Cholesterol	0 mg
Dietary Fiber	.855 g
Total Vitamin A	.631 RE
A–Retinol	0 RE
A–Carotenoid	.631 RE
Thiamin–B1	.025 mg
Riboflavin–B2	.012 mg
Niacin–B3	.399 mg
Niacin Equivalent	.399 mg
Vitamin B6	.026 mg
Vitamin B12	0 mcg
Folate	3.61 mcg
Pantothenic	.113 mg
Vitamin C	.025 mg
Vitamin D	0 mcg
Vitamin E-Alpha E	.148 mg

Calcium	4.2 mg
Copper	.051 mg
Iron	.166 mg
Magnesium	7.24 mg
Manganese	.112 mg
Phosphorus	12.2 mg
Potassium	75.2 mg
Selenium	.343 mcg
Sodium	.376 mg
Zinc	.14 mg
Complex Carbohydrates	.213 g
Sugars	6.39 g
Mono-Saccharide	0 g
Di-Saccharide	4.26 g
Alcohol	0 g
Caffeine	0 mg
Water	2.21 g

⊚ Sweet Almonds

Calories	26.3
Protein	.744 g
Carbohydrates	.674 g
Fat—Total	2.47 g
Saturated Fat	.287 g
Monounsaturated Fat	1.5 g
Polyunsaturated Fat	.578 g
Omega 3 Fatty Acid	.016 g
Omega 6 Fatty Acid	.561 g
Cholesterol	0 mg
Dietary Fiber	.353 g
Total Vitamin A	7.05 RE
A–Retinol	6.45 RE
A–Carotenoid	.58 RE
Thiamin–B1	.006 mg
Riboflavin–B2	.025 mg
Niacin–B3	.115 mg
Niacin Equivalent	.115 mg
Vitamin B6	.004 mg
Vitamin B12	0 mcg
Folate	1.4 mcg
Pantothenic	.017 mg
Vitamin C	.022 mg
Vitamin D	0 mcg
Vitamin E-Alpha E	.294 mg

Calcium	9.07 mg
Copper	.039 mg
Iron	.132 mg
Magnesium	10.4 mg
Manganese	.052 mg
Phosphorus	19.4 mg
Potassium	27.4 mg
Selenium	.171 mcg
Sodium	.378 mg
Zinc	.115 mg
Complex Carbohydrates	.116 g
Sugars	.207 g
Mono-Saccharide	0 g
Di-Saccharide	0 g
Alcohol	0 g
Caffeine	0 mg
Water	.328 g

◉ Sweet Fruit

Calories	18.4
Protein	.338 g
Carbohydrates	3.19 g
Fat—Total	.661 g
Saturated Fat	.129 g
Monounsaturated Fat	.385 g
Polyunsaturated Fat	.113 g
Omega 3 Fatty Acid	.003 g
Omega 6 Fatty Acid	.11 g
Cholesterol	0 mg
Dietary Fiber	.329 g
Total Vitamin A	8.57 RE
A–Retinol	0 RE
A–Carotenoid	8.57 RE
Thiamin–B1	.007 mg
Riboflavin–B2	.008 mg
Niacin–B3	.085 mg
Niacin Equivalent	.085 mg
Vitamin B6	.014 mg
Vitamin B12	0 mcg
Folate	1.21 mcg
Pantothenic	.031 mg
Vitamin C	.278 mg
Vitamin D	0 mcg
Vitamin E-Alpha E	.062 mg

Calcium	2.7 mg
Copper	.046 mg
Iron	.177 mg
Magnesium	5.18 mg
Manganese	.022 mg
Phosphorus	10.2 mg
Potassium	40.1 mg
Selenium	.497 mcg
Sodium	.499 mg
Zinc	.097 mg
Complex Carbohydrates	.309 g
Sugars	2.3 g
Mono-Saccharide	1.82 g
Di-Saccharide	.196 g
Alcohol	0 g
Caffeine	0 mg
Water	2.32 g

❾ Sweet Nuts

Calories	6.51
Protein	.143 g
Carbohydrates	.184 g
Fat—Total	.619 g
Saturated Fat	.056 g
Monounsaturated Fat	.142 g
Polyunsaturated Fat	.391 g
Omega 3 Fatty Acid	.068 g
Omega 6 Fatty Acid	.318 g
Cholesterol	0 mg
Dietary Fiber	.045 g
Total Vitamin A	.124 RE
A–Retinol	0 RE
A–Carotenoid	.124 RE
Thiamin–B1	.004 mg
Riboflavin–B2	.001 mg
Niacin–B3	.01 mg
Niacin Equivalent	.01 mg
Vitamin B6	.006 mg
Vitamin B12	0 mcg
Folate	.66 mcg
Pantothenic	.006 mg
Vitamin C	.032 mg
Vitamin D	0 mcg
Vitamin E-Alpha E	.026 mg

Calcium	.941 mg
Copper	.014 mg
Iron	.025 mg
Magnesium	1.69 mg
Manganese	.029 mg
Phosphorus	3.17 mg
Potassium	5.02 mg
Selenium	.05 mcg
Sodium	.101 mg
Zinc	.027 mg
Complex Carbohydrates	.117 g
Sugars	.022 g
Mono-Saccharide	0 g
Di-Saccharide	.021 g
Alcohol	0 g
Caffeine	0 mg
Water	.063 g

☉ Sweet Sesame

Calories	68
Protein	2.39 g
Carbohydrates	3.95 g
Fat—Total	5.38 g
Saturated Fat	.693 g
Monounsaturated Fat	1.84 g
Polyunsaturated Fat	2.6 g
Omega 3 Fatty Acid	.17 g
Omega 6 Fatty Acid	2.42 g
Cholesterol	0 mg
Dietary Fiber	.897 g
Total Vitamin A	.775 RE
A–Retinol	0 RE
A–Carotenoid	.775 RE
Thiamin–B1	.067 mg
Riboflavin–B2	.013 mg
Niacin–B3	.402 mg
Niacin Equivalent	.403 mg
Vitamin B6	.031 mg
Vitamin B12	0 mcg
Folate	8.66 mcg
Pantothenic	.065 mg
Vitamin C	.185 mg
Vitamin D	0 mcg
Vitamin E-Alpha E	.266 mg

Calcium	13.5 mg
Copper	.149 mg
Iron	.71 mg
Magnesium	30.7 mg
Manganese	.177 mg
Phosphorus	68.1 mg
Potassium	67.9 mg
Selenium	.943 mcg
Sodium	3.64 mg
Zinc	.84 mg
Complex Carbohydrates	.344 g
Sugars	2.85 g
Mono-Saccharide	2.36 g
Di-Saccharide	.042 g
Alcohol	0 g
Caffeine	0 mg
Water	.994 g

⑨ Sweet Snack

Calories	60.2
Protein	1.54 g
Carbohydrates	5.78 g
Fat—Total	3.81 g
Saturated Fat	1.46 g
Monounsaturated Fat	.915 g
Polyunsaturated Fat	1.18 g
Omega 3 Fatty Acid	.137 g
Omega 6 Fatty Acid	1.03 g
Cholesterol	.302 mg
Dietary Fiber	.461 g
Total Vitamin A	.634 RE
A–Retinol	0 RE
A–Carotenoid	.39 RE
Thiamin–B1	.023 mg
Riboflavin–B2	.008 mg
Niacin–B3	.38 mg
Niacin Equivalent	.38 mg
Vitamin B6	.027 mg
Vitamin B12	0 mcg
Folate	5.15 mcg
Pantothenic	.057 mg
Vitamin C	.241 mg
Vitamin D	0 mcg
Vitamin E-Alpha E	.25 mg

Calcium	28.6 mg
Copper	.055 mg
Iron	.208 mg
Magnesium	9.61 mg
Manganese	.14 mg
Phosphorus	18.3 mg
Potassium	52.4 mg
Selenium	.441 mcg
Sodium	.728 mg
Zinc	.153 mg
Complex Carbohydrates	.657 g
Sugars	3.87 g
Mono-Saccharide	1.58 g
Di-Saccharide	.139 g
Alcohol	0 g
Caffeine	0 mg
Water	.549 g

☉ Trail Mix

Calories	30.6
Protein	.876 g
Carbohydrates	3.83 g
Fat—Total	1.5 g
Saturated Fat	.36 g
Monounsaturated Fat	.655 g
Polyunsaturated Fat	.384 g
Omega 3 Fatty Acid	.001 g
Omega 6 Fatty Acid	.382 g
Cholesterol	.07 mg
Dietary Fiber	.274 g
Total Vitamin A	.074 RE
A–Retinol	0 RE
A–Carotenoid	.018 RE
Thiamin–B1	.022 mg
Riboflavin–B2	.011 mg
Niacin–B3	.402 mg
Niacin Equivalent	.402 mg
Vitamin B6	.012 mg
Vitamin B12	0 mcg
Folate	3.81 mcg
Pantothenic	.039 mg
Vitamin C	.074 mg
Vitamin D	0 mcg
Vitamin E-Alpha E	.19 mg

Calcium	9.66 mg
Copper	.025 mg
Iron	.189 mg
Magnesium	5.09 mg
Manganese	.064 mg
Phosphorus	11.8 mg
Potassium	42.7 mg
Selenium	.495 mcg
Sodium	10.2 mg
Zinc	.092 mg
Complex Carbohydrates	1.26 g
Sugars	2.1 g
Mono-Saccharide	1.46 g
Di-Saccharide	.09 g
Alcohol	0 g
Caffeine	0 mg
Water	.441 g

⊚ Truffles

Calories	57.2
Protein	1.88 g
Carbohydrates	5.88 g
Fat—Total	3.02 g
Saturated Fat	2.06 g
Monounsaturated Fat	.401 g
Polyunsaturated Fat	.254 g
Omega 3 Fatty Acid	0 g
Omega 6 Fatty Acid	.254 g
Cholesterol	.806 mg
Dietary Fiber	.112 g
Total Vitamin A	.648 RE
A–Retinol	0 RE
A–Carotenoid	0 RE
Thiamin–B1	.007 mg
Riboflavin–B2	.002 mg
Niacin–B3	.219 mg
Niacin Equivalent	.219 mg
Vitamin B6	.004 mg
Vitamin B12	0 mcg
Folate	2.36 mcg
Pantothenic	.023 mg
Vitamin C	0 mg
Vitamin D	0 mcg
Vitamin E-Alpha E	.12 mg

Calcium	64.6 mg
Copper	.011 mg
Iron	.128 mg
Magnesium	2.84 mg
Manganese	.034 mg
Phosphorus	5.81 mg
Potassium	10.7 mg
Selenium	.12 mcg
Sodium	.097 mg
Zinc	.054 mg
Complex Carbohydrates	.162 g
Sugars	3.54 g
Mono-Saccharide	.003 g
Di-Saccharide	.065 g
Alcohol	0 g
Caffeine	0 mg
Water	.025 g

◉ Vanilla Cake

Calories	47.8
Protein	1.21 g
Carbohydrates	5.15 g
Fat—Total	2.53 g
Saturated Fat	.34 g
Monounsaturated Fat	1.24 g
Polyunsaturated Fat	.833 g
Omega 3 Fatty Acid	.016 g
Omega 6 Fatty Acid	.816 g
Cholesterol	0 mg
Dietary Fiber	.302 g
Total Vitamin A	35.2 RE
A–Retinol	32.2 RE
A–Carotenoid	2.9 RE
Thiamin–B1	.058 mg
Riboflavin–B2	.055 mg
Niacin–B3	.481 mg
Niacin Equivalent	.482 mg
Vitamin B6	.005 mg
Vitamin B12	.007 mcg
Folate	2.48 mcg
Pantothenic	.042 mg
Vitamin C	.016 mg
Vitamin D	.377 mcg
Vitamin E-Alpha E	.73 mg

Calcium	7.24 mg
Copper	.028 mg
Iron	.518 mg
Magnesium	7.56 mg
Manganese	.086 mg
Phosphorus	16.9 mg
Potassium	26.4 mg
Selenium	.861 mcg
Sodium	17.2 mg
Zinc	.099 mg
Complex Carbohydrates	4.59 g
Sugars	.262 g
Mono-Saccharide	.028 g
Di-Saccharide	.11 g
Alcohol	0 g
Caffeine	0 mg
Water	5.24 g

⊚ Vanilla Drops

Calories	28.4
Protein	.449 g
Carbohydrates	3.2 g
Fat—Total	1.51 g
Saturated Fat	.249 g
Monounsaturated Fat	.553 g
Polyunsaturated Fat	.633 g
Omega 3 Fatty Acid	.008 g
Omega 6 Fatty Acid	.627 g
Cholesterol	0 mg
Dietary Fiber	.136 g
Total Vitamin A	37.6 RE
A–Retinol	34.4 RE
A–Carotenoid	3.09 RE
Thiamin–B1	.033 mg
Riboflavin–B2	.021 mg
Niacin–B3	.247 mg
Niacin Equivalent	.247 mg
Vitamin B6	.002 mg
Vitamin B12	.002 mcg
Folate	1.11 mcg
Pantothenic	.02 mg
Vitamin C	.004 mg
Vitamin D	.403 mcg
Vitamin E-Alpha E	.25 mg

Calcium	1.3 mg
Copper	.006 mg
Iron	.194 mg
Magnesium	.976 mg
Manganese	.028 mg
Phosphorus	5.02 mg
Potassium	5.42 mg
Selenium	1.41 mcg
Sodium	13.4 mg
Zinc	.029 mg
Complex Carbohydrates	2.97 g
Sugars	.088 g
Mono-Saccharide	.038 g
Di-Saccharide	.017 g
Alcohol	0 g
Caffeine	0 mg
Water	2.74 g

⑨ Vanilla Raisin Clusters

Calories	32.5
Protein	.718 g
Carbohydrates	5.91 g
Fat—Total	.854 g
Saturated Fat	.738 g
Monounsaturated Fat	.001 g
Polyunsaturated Fat	.007 g
Omega 3 Fatty Acid	.002 g
Omega 6 Fatty Acid	.005 g
Cholesterol	.302 mg
Dietary Fiber	.168 g
Total Vitamin A	.282 RE
A–Retinol	0 RE
A–Carotenoid	.039 RE
Thiamin–B1	.008 mg
Riboflavin–B2	.004 mg
Niacin–B3	.04 mg
Niacin Equivalent	.04 mg
Vitamin B6	.012 mg
Vitamin B12	0 mcg
Folate	.16 mcg
Pantothenic	.002 mg
Vitamin C	.16 mg
Vitamin D	0 mcg
Vitamin E-Alpha E	.034 mg

Calcium	26.3 mg
Copper	.015 mg
Iron	.135 mg
Magnesium	1.6 mg
Manganese	.015 mg
Phosphorus	4.7 mg
Potassium	36.3 mg
Selenium	.322 mcg
Sodium	.581 mg
Zinc	.013 mg
Complex Carbohydrates	0 g
Sugars	4.94 g
Mono-Saccharide	3.14 g
Di-Saccharide	0 g
Alcohol	0 g
Caffeine	0 mg
Water	.788 g

⑨ Walnut Fudge

Calories	137
Protein	3.72 g
Carbohydrates	13.5 g
Fat—Total	7.97 g
Saturated Fat	3.57 g
Monounsaturated Fat	1.15 g
Polyunsaturated Fat	2.63 g
Omega 3 Fatty Acid	.464 g
Omega 6 Fatty Acid	2.14 g
Cholesterol	3.94 mg
Dietary Fiber	.302 g
Total Vitamin A	8.44 RE
A–Retinol	6.03 RE
A–Carotenoid	1.49 RE
Thiamin–B1	.033 mg
Riboflavin–B2	.044 mg
Niacin–B3	.087 mg
Niacin Equivalent	.087 mg
Vitamin B6	.041 mg
Vitamin B12	.037 mcg
Folate	5.33 mcg
Pantothenic	.104 mg
Vitamin C	.43 mg
Vitamin D	.01 mcg
Vitamin E-Alpha E	.192 mg

Calcium	119 mg
Copper	.094 mg
Iron	.308 mg
Magnesium	13.4 mg
Manganese	.194 mg
Phosphorus	42 mg
Potassium	64.1 mg
Selenium	.418 mcg
Sodium	11.2 mg
Zinc	.261 mg
Complex Carbohydrates	.779 g
Sugars	9.51 g
Mono-Saccharide	0 g
Di-Saccharide	4.63 g
Alcohol	0 g
Caffeine	0 mg
Water	2.57 g

⑨ White Frosting

Calories	234
Protein	35.5 g
Carbohydrates	12.6 g
Fat—Total	.11 g
Saturated Fat	.071 g
Monounsaturated Fat	.03 g
Polyunsaturated Fat	.003 g
Omega 3 Fatty Acid	.001 g
Omega 6 Fatty Acid	.002 g
Cholesterol	41 mg
Dietary Fiber	0 g
Total Vitamin A	638 RE
A–Retinol	1.2 RE
A–Carotenoid	.031 RE
Thiamin–B1	.029 mg
Riboflavin–B2	.599 mg
Niacin–B3	.076 mg
Niacin Equivalent	.077 mg
Vitamin B6	.032 mg
Vitamin B12	.375 mcg
Folate	7.48 mcg
Pantothenic	.393 mg
Vitamin C	.532 mg
Vitamin D	.025 mcg
Vitamin E-Alpha E	.003 mg

Calcium	123 mg
Copper	.009 mg
Iron	.055 mg
Magnesium	11.7 mg
Manganese	.003 mg
Phosphorus	96.3 mg
Potassium	156 mg
Selenium	2.16 mcg
Sodium	1406 mg
Zinc	.595 mg
Complex Carbohydrates	0 g
Sugars	4.7 g
Mono-Saccharide	0 g
Di-Saccharide	0 g
Alcohol	0 g
Caffeine	0 mg
Water	52.2 g

⑨ Yummy Bananas

Calories	54.6
Protein	1.63 g
Carbohydrates	6.89 g
Fat—Total	2.37 g
Saturated Fat	2.07 g
Monounsaturated Fat	.002 g
Polyunsaturated Fat	.004 g
Omega 3 Fatty Acid	.001 g
Omega 6 Fatty Acid	.002 g
Cholesterol	.854 mg
Dietary Fiber	.09 g
Total Vitamin A	1.05 RE
A–Retinol	0 RE
A–Carotenoid	.359 RE
Thiamin–B1	.002 mg
Riboflavin–B2	.003 mg
Niacin–B3	.033 mg
Niacin Equivalent	.033 mg
Vitamin B6	.006 mg
Vitamin B12	0 mcg
Folate	.471 mcg
Pantothenic	.003 mg
Vitamin C	.082 mg
Vitamin D	0 mcg
Vitamin E-Alpha E	.012 mg

Calcium	67.8 mg
Copper	.005 mg
Iron	.11 mg
Magnesium	1.27 mg
Manganese	.007 mg
Phosphorus	.871 mg
Potassium	17.5 mg
Selenium	.032 mcg
Sodium	.035 mg
Zinc	.007 mg
Complex Carbohydrates	.255 g
Sugars	4.36 g
Mono-Saccharide	0 g
Di-Saccharide	0 g
Alcohol	0 g
Caffeine	0 mg
Water	.035 g

Index